A 30-Day Chia Seed Cleanse

Constipation-Free Living

Alice Klayn

DISCLAIMER **5**

INTRODUCTION **6**

CHAPTER 1: UNDERSTANDING CONSTIPATION.................................. **8**

THE POWER OF CHIA SEEDS FOR CONSTIPATION 12

CONSTIPATION CONTROL WITH CHIA SEEDS WILL HELP YOU 16

CHAPTER 2: CHIA SEEDS AND POWERFUL NUTRITION.............. **21**

NUTRITIONAL PROFILE OF CHIA SEEDS 25

HOW CHIA SEEDS AID DIGESTION.. 29

**CHAPTER 3: PREPARING FOR THE CLEANSE OF THE BODY
WITH CHIA SEEDS**.. **34**

SETTING YOUR GOALS AND EXPECTATIONS FOR CONSTIPATION MANAGEMENT ... 38

ESSENTIAL INGREDIENTS FOR USING CHIA SEEDS TO COMBAT CONSTIPATION..... 41

CHAPTER 4: WEEK 1 - STARTING THE JOURNEY........................... **46**

USING CHIA SEEDS... **46**

DAILY MEAL PLANS AND RECIPES WITH CHIA SEEDS FOR CONSTIPATION............ 49

DEFINING THE BEST TIMES TO USE CHIA SEEDS TO CONTROL CONSTIPATION 54

**CHAPTER 5: WEEK 2 - DEEPENING THE CLEANSE OF THE BODY
WITH CHIA SEEDS**... **59**

PRACTICAL AND EFFECTIVE RECIPES WITH CHIA SEEDS FOR CONSTIPATION.......... 62

DEALING WITH DETOX SYMPTOMS WITH CHIA SEEDS 66

**CHAPTER 6: WEEK 3 - MAXIMIZING BENEFITS WITH CHIA
SEEDS**.. **72**

OPTIMIZING YOUR CHIA SEED INTAKE 76

INCORPORATING HEALTHY HABITS FOR CONSTIPATION MANAGEMENT............... 79

**CHAPTER 7: WEEK 4 - SUPPORTING CLEANSING FOR
CONSTIPATION CONTROL WITH CHIA SEEDS**.................................. **83**

MAINTAINING TRANSFORMATIONAL MOMENTUM FOR CONSTIPATION CONTROL
WITH CHIA SEEDS 87

TRANSITIONING TO LONG-TERM HEALTH OF THE BODY WITH CHIA SEEDS 91

**CHAPTER 8: LIFESTYLE TIPS FOR REGULARITY OF
CONSTIPATION CONTROL**... **96**

Specific Exercise and Physical Activity to Reduce Constipation 99
Stress Management and Sleep 104

CHAPTER 9: LONG-TERM HEALTH AND WELLNESS 109

Creating a Sustainable Routine 112
Celebrating Your Success in Reducing Constipation with Chia Seeds .. 116

CHAPTER 10: CHIA SEEDS AND HYDRATION 120

Importance of Staying Hydrated for Constipation Control 123
How Chia Seeds Help with Body Hydration 127

CONCLUSION 130

BIOGRAPHY 132

BONUS 01: CHIA-INFUSED-DRINKS-HYDRATING 134

BONUS 02: CHIA-SEEDS-FOR-CONSTIPATION-RECIPE 134

BONUS 03: CHIA-SEED-SMOOTHIES-FOR-CONSTIPATION 134

GLOSSARY: CHIA SEEDS FOR CONSTIPATION 135

Disclaimer

The information provided in "A 30-Day Chia Seed Cleanse: Constipation-Free Living" by Alice Klayn is for educational and informational purposes only.

Always seek the advice of your physician or other qualified health provider with any questions you may have regarding a medical condition.

While every effort has been made to ensure the accuracy of the information contained in this book, the author and publisher assume no responsibility for errors, omissions, or contrary interpretation of the subject matter herein.

The content is based on personal research, experiences, and insights and should not be considered a definitive guide.

Introduction

Welcome to "**A 30-Day Chia Seed Cleanse: Constipation-Free Living**"—your ultimate guide to harnessing the power of chia seeds for a healthier, happier digestive system. If you've been struggling with constipation and are searching for a natural, effective solution, you've come to the right place. This book is designed to transform your life by providing you with a simple yet powerful tool: chia seeds.

Chia seeds are more than just a trendy superfood; they are a potent remedy for digestive issues that have been used for centuries. Packed with fiber, omega-3 fatty acids, and essential nutrients, these tiny seeds are your ticket to a constipation-free life. In this book, we'll guide you through a 30-day journey that will not only alleviate your constipation but also revitalize your overall health.

Learn about the hidden nutritional power within these tiny seeds and why they are so effective in promoting digestive health. Enjoy delicious, easy-to-make recipes that incorporate chia seeds into every meal, ensuring you receive their full benefits without compromising on taste.

Discover practical advice on how to incorporate chia seeds into your daily routine, along with lifestyle tips to enhance your digestive health. Be inspired by real-life testimonials from people who have transformed their lives through the 30-Day Chia Seed Cleanse.

By the end of this 30-day cleanse, you will not only

experience relief from constipation but also a newfound sense of vitality and well-being. Embrace the journey, trust the process, and get ready to feel lighter, healthier, and more energized than ever before. Let's embark on this transformative journey together and discover the incredible benefits of chia seeds for constipation-free living.

Chapter 1: Understanding Constipation

Although it can be uncomfortable and frustrating, understanding the underlying mechanisms of constipation empowers individuals to make informed decisions about their health and well-being. This chapter aims to provide a comprehensive overview of constipation, including its definitions, causes, symptoms, and potential treatments.

What is Constipation?

Constipation is typically defined as infrequent bowel movements or difficult-to-pass stools. While the frequency of bowel movements can vary widely from person to person, having fewer than three bowel movements per week is commonly accepted as constipation. However, this definition often overlooks the nuances of the condition, as irregularity, stool hardness, and the effort required to pass stools are crucial aspects of the constipation experience.

Normal Bowel Function

To understand constipation, it's essential first to understand normal bowel function. The digestive system is designed to process food and eliminate waste efficiently. The large intestine, or colon, plays a critical role in this process:

Waste Formation: As food moves through the digestive tract, nutrients are absorbed in the small intestine, while the remaining waste is transferred to the colon. Here, water is reabsorbed, and the waste is compacted into stool.

Muscle Contractions: The colon is lined with smooth muscles that contract rhythmically to propel the stool towards the rectum. This process, known as peristalsis, is vital for maintaining regular bowel habits.

Nerve Signals: The nervous system, including the enteric nervous system (sometimes called the "second brain"), plays a significant role in regulating bowel movements. It coordinates the complex interaction of muscles and sphincters, allowing for effective elimination.

Causes of Constipation

Constipation can arise from various factors, often interacting in complex ways. Some of the most common causes include:

1. Dietary Factors

A diet low in fiber is one of the primary contributors to constipation. Fiber, found in fruits, vegetables, whole grains, and legumes, adds bulk to the stool and helps retain water, making it easier to pass. Conversely, diets high in processed foods, which tend to be low in fiber, can lead to hard, dry stools.

2. Dehydration

Water is vital for digestion and stool formation. Insufficient fluid intake can result in harder stools, makingthem more challenging to pass.

3. Sedentary Lifestyle

Physical activity promotes bowel health by stimulating

peristalsis. Sedentary individuals may experience slower bowel movements and a higher incidence of constipation.

4. Medications

Certain medications, including painkillers, antacids containing aluminum, and some antidepressants, can contribute to constipation as a side effect. Individuals on these medications should consult their healthcareprovider if they experience changes in bowel habits.

5. Medical Conditions

Several medical conditions can predispose individuals to constipation. These include:

Hypothyroidism: An underactive thyroid can slow down metabolism, leading to sluggish bowelmovements.

Diabetes: High blood sugar levels can damage nerves that control bowel function, leading toconstipation.

Irritable Bowel Syndrome (IBS): This digestive disorder often presents with alternating patterns of constipation and diarrhea.

Neurological Disorders: Conditions such as Parkinson's disease, multiple sclerosis, and spinal cord injuries can affect nerve function and bowel control.

6. Psychological Factors

Psychological issues, including stress, anxiety, and

depression, may impact bowel habits. The gut-brain axis—the communication pathway between the digestive system and the brain—plays a significant role in regulating gastrointestinal function.

7. Lifestyle Factors

Ignoring the urge to have a bowel movement, which can occur due to distractions, busy schedules, or discomfort, may lead to constipation. This behavior teaches the body to suppress the urge over time.

Symptoms of Constipation

The symptoms of constipation can vary in severity and may include:

Infrequent bowel movements (fewer than three times a week)
Hard, dry stools
Straining during bowel movements
A feeling of incomplete evacuation
Abdominal discomfort or bloating

While these symptoms are common, chronic constipation—defined as constipation lasting more than three months—can significantly affect an individual's quality of life, leading to emotional stress and physical discomfort.

Understanding constipation is pivotal for addressing the condition effectively. By recognizing its causes and symptoms, individuals can take proactive measures to improve their bowel health.

The Power of Chia Seeds for Constipation

Characterized by infrequent bowel movements, difficulty in passing stools, and general feelings of discomfort, chronic constipation can significantly impair quality of life. While various dietary and lifestyle changes can help alleviate this condition, one superfood has garnered attention for its potential benefits: chia seeds. In this chapter, we will explore the science behind chia seeds, their nutritional profile, and how they can be effectively incorporated into a diet to promote regular bowel movements and improve digestive health.

Understanding Constipation

Before delving into the benefits of chia seeds, it's essential to understand what causes constipation. A range of factors can contribute to this condition, including a low-fiber diet, inadequate hydration, stress, lack of physical activity, and certain medications or medical conditions. In many cases, incorporating more fiber into the diet can help address these issues by promoting regular bowel movements and enhancing overall gut health.

The Nutritional Profile of Chia Seeds

Chia seeds are tiny black or white seeds from the Salvia hispanica plant, native to Central America. Despite their small size, chia seeds are packed with essential nutrients that make them a powerhouse of health benefits:

High Fiber Content: Chia seeds are an excellent source of dietary fiber, with approximately 11 grams of fiber per ounce (about two tablespoons). This high fiber content can facilitate bowel movements by adding bulk to the stool and promoting regularity.

Hydrophilic Properties: One of the unique characteristics of chia seeds is their ability to absorb liquid. When soaked in water or another liquid, chia seeds can expand up to 10-12 times their weight, forming a gel-like consistency. This gel can help soften stools, making them easier to pass.

Omega-3 Fatty Acids: Chia seeds are rich in alpha-linolenic acid (ALA), a type of omega-3 fatty acid. These healthy fats can contribute to overall well-being, including supporting gut health and reducing inflammation in the digestive tract.

Antioxidants: Chia seeds are loaded with antioxidants, which help combat oxidative stress and inflammation in the body, promoting overall health and potentially supporting a healthy gut environment.

Essential Minerals: Chia seeds are a good source of several important minerals, including calcium, magnesium, and phosphorus, which are vital for maintaining bone health and overall bodily functions.

How Chia Seeds Alleviate Constipation #### 1. **Increased Fiber Intake**

The most direct way in which chia seeds can help with constipation is through their fiber content. Dietary fiber plays a crucial role in digestive health by adding bulk to stools and facilitating their passage through the intestines. Regularly consuming chia seeds can significantly increase your daily fiber intake, contributing to improved bowel regularity.

2. **Hydration and Gel Formation**

When chia seeds are mixed with liquid, they swell and form a gel. Consuming this gel not only adds moisture to the digestive system but also helps to soften stools. This gel-like consistency can make stools easier to pass, reducing the discomfort associated with constipation.

3. **Promoting Healthy Gut Flora**

A healthy gut microbiome is essential for regular bowel movements. The fiber in chia seeds acts as a prebiotic, providing nourishment for beneficial gut bacteria. A healthy balance of gut flora can improve digestive health and may alleviate the symptoms of constipation.

4. **Regulating Bowel Movements**

The combination of soluble and insoluble fiber in chia seeds helps to regulate bowel movements. Soluble fiber dissolves in water to form a gel, while insoluble fiber adds bulk to the stool. This balance supports the natural function of the digestive system, encouraging regularity.

Incorporating Chia Seeds into Your Diet

Adding chia seeds to your daily diet is simple and versatile. Here are some easy ways to incorporate them:

Chia Pudding: Combine chia seeds with your choice of milk (or a dairy-free alternative), sweetener, and flavorings such as vanilla or cocoa powder. Let it sit overnight in the refrigerator to create a delicious pudding.

Smoothies: Blend chia seeds into your favorite smoothie for an added nutrient boost. They canenhance the thickness and texture of the smoothie while contributing to your fiber intake.

Baked Goods: Add chia seeds to muffins, bread, and other baked goods. They can replace eggs in recipes, providing a binding effect when mixed with water.

Sprinkled on Salads: Toss chia seeds onto salads, yogurt, or oatmeal for a nutritional boost that adds a pleasant crunch.

Soups and Stews: Stir chia seeds into soups or stews as a thickening agent, which can enhance thetexture and fiber content of the dish.

Chia seeds are not only a trendy superfood but also a powerful ally in combating constipation. By enhancing your fiber intake, contributing to gut health, and promoting regular bowel movements, chia seeds can play an essential role in your diet. Whether consumed in puddings, smoothies, baked goods, or sprinkled on meals, incorporating these tiny seeds can lead to significant improvements in digestive health.

Constipation Control with Chia Seeds Will Help You

While occasional constipation may not be a major concern, chronic constipation can lead to significant discomfort and may even signal underlying health problems. Traditionally, many have turned to laxatives or over-the-counter remedies to relieve their symptoms. However, there is a gentler, more natural approach that has gained considerable attention: a 30-day cleanse utilizing the remarkable benefits of chia seeds.

The Constipation Challenge

To understand the efficacy of a 30-day cleanse with chia seeds, it's essential to comprehend what causes constipation. Factors contributing to this condition may include a diet low in fiber, inadequate hydration, lack of physical activity, and certain medications or medical conditions. An imbalance in gut bacteria and a stressful lifestyle can also play crucial roles in digestive health. Thus, addressing constipation effectively often requires a multifaceted approach that targets diet, hydration, exercise, and stress management.

Enter Chia Seeds: The Superfood

Chia seeds, tiny black seeds derived from the Salvia hispanica plant, have been praised as a superfood due to their rich nutritional profile. These seeds are packed with omega-3 fatty acids, protein, antioxidants, and most importantly, soluble and insoluble fiber. This combination of nutrients offers numerous health benefits, particularly for digestive health.

One ounce (28 grams) of chia seeds contains about 11 grams of dietary fiber—vastly exceeding the fiber content of many everyday foods. The unique ability of chia seeds to absorb water and expand in the stomach also plays a crucial role in their effectiveness as a natural remedy for constipation.

How a 30-Day Cleanse Works

The premise of a 30-day cleanse is to reset your digestive system by incorporating nutrient-dense foods that promote gut health while eliminating processed foods and potential irritants. During this month, chia seeds serve as a core component of your diet, helping to facilitate regular bowel movements and improve overall digestive function.

Week 1: Introduction and Adaptation

In the first week, the focus is on integrating chia seeds into your diet. Begin with small amounts—about one tablespoon daily. Chia seeds can be easily added to smoothies, yogurt, oatmeal, or salads. This week is all about allowing your body to adjust to the increased fiber intake while eliminating foods that can exacerbate constipation, such as white bread, sugary snacks, and processed foods.

Week 2: Building Fiber Intake

As your body adapts, increase your chia seed intake to two tablespoons daily while continuing to eliminate constipating foods. Support your digestive system by increasing your intake of water. Chia seeds can absorbup to 12 times their weight in water, and adequate hydration is crucial to ensure that the fiber can do its job effectively without causing bloating or discomfort.

Week 3: Focus on Gut Health

In the third week, begin incorporating other fibrous foods—such as fruits, vegetables, and whole grains—while maintaining your chia seed consumption. This combination will not only keep your digestion moving smoothly but also support the growth of healthy gut bacteria. The soluble fiber from chia seeds helpsto create a gel-like substance in the gut, which can facilitate the smooth passage of stool.

Week 4: Maintenance and Reflection

As you enter the final week of your cleanse, reflect on how your body has responded. Are you experiencing more regular bowel movements? Is your bloating or discomfort subsiding? Continue with your chia seed intake, aiming for around three tablespoons a day, and keep hydrating. This final week is about solidifying new habits that keep your gut health in check beyond the 30 days.

The Benefits of the 30-Day Cleanse

The benefits of a 30-day cleanse using chia seeds extend far beyond just alleviating constipation. Participants often report increased energy levels, clearer skin, greater appetite control, and improved mood—all of which can be attributed to a cleaner diet and healthier digestion.

Enhanced Digestion: The soluble and insoluble fiber found in chia seeds works synergistically to support gut health, promote regularity, and prevent constipation.

Increased Hydration: With chia seeds' unique ability to absorb water, the cleanse encourages higher fluid intake, which is essential for digestive health.

Sustained Energy: A fiber-rich diet helps stabilize blood sugar levels, preventing the spikes and crashes associated with a typical high-sugar diet.

Nutrient-Rich: Chia seeds are packed with essential nutrients that can enhance overall health, including vitamins, minerals, and antioxidants.

Holistic Approach: The cleanse incorporates not just dietary changes but also emphasizes the importance of hydration, physical activity, and stress management—crucial factors in maintaining good digestive health.

A 30-day cleanse for constipation control with chia seeds is not just a quick fix; it's an investment in your health and well-being. By committing to this transformative journey, you'll learn the importance of mindful eating and hydration while developing habits that can support a healthy digestive system long after the cleanse is complete.

Chapter 2: Chia Seeds and powerful nutrition

Tiny yet powerful, these small seeds are nutritional powerhouses that have captivated health enthusiasts and nutritionists alike. By exploring the world of chia seeds, we uncover their origins, nutritional profile, and the numerous ways they can enhance our overall health and well-being.

The Origins of Chia Seeds

Chia seeds (Salvia hispanica) trace their roots back to the ancient Aztec and Mayan civilizations, where they were esteemed for their energy-boosting properties. The word "chia" means "strength" in the Mayan language, reflecting their significant impact on stamina and overall health. Historically, warriors consumed these seeds before battle to boost their endurance and vitality.

Today, chia seeds have moved beyond their ancient origins to become a global health and wellness staple. They are primarily grown in Mexico and South America, thriving in sunny climates and well-drained soils. Their modern popularity is due to their impressive health benefits and versatile culinary uses.

Nutritional Powerhouse

Chia seeds are often hailed as a superfood because of their exceptional nutrient density. These tiny seeds are packed with essential nutrients, making them a valuable addition to any diet. A typical serving of chia seeds (about 28 grams or two tablespoons) offers an impressive array of nutrients:

Omega-3 Fatty Acids: Chia seeds are one of the richest plant-based sources of omega-3 fatty acids, particularly alpha-linolenic acid (ALA). Omega-3s are essential for heart health, reducing inflammation, and supporting brain function.

Fiber: With approximately 10 grams of dietary fiber per serving, chia seeds promote digestive health, help maintain a healthy weight, and regulate blood sugar levels.

Protein: Each serving of chia seeds contains around 4 grams of protein, providing a good plant-based protein source necessary for muscle repair and growth, satiety, and overall bodily functions.

Minerals: Chia seeds are rich in vital minerals such as calcium, magnesium, phosphorus, and potassium, which are crucial for bone health, muscle function, and maintaining healthy blood pressure levels.

Antioxidants: Chia seeds contain antioxidants that help combat oxidative stress and may reduce the risk of chronic diseases. These compounds also contribute to the seeds' long shelf life and nutritional stability.

Hydration: When soaked in water or liquid, chia seeds form a gel-like substance due to their unique soluble fiber content. This property aids in hydration and creates a feeling of fullness, making them an excellent ally in weight management.

Chia seeds offer a remarkable blend of nutrients that support various aspects of health, making them a powerful addition to any diet.

Health Benefits of Chia Seeds

Incorporating chia seeds into your diet offers numerous health benefits that can support both physical and mental wellbeing. Here are some of the key advantages:

Heart Health

The high omega-3 fatty acid content in chia seeds has a positive impact on heart health. Regular consumption can help lower bad cholesterol (LDL) levels and raise good cholesterol (HDL) levels, thereby reducing the risk of heart disease. Additionally, the fiber in chia seeds contributes to healthy cholesterol levels and blood pressure regulation.

Digestive Health

Chia seeds are a natural source of fiber, which aids digestion and promotes regular bowel movements. The soluble fiber in chia seeds absorbs water, swelling to create a gel-like consistency that helps move food through the digestive tract smoothly. This can alleviate issues such as constipation and bloating.

Weight Management

Including chia seeds in your meals can enhance feelings of satiety and reduce the urge to snack between meals. Their ability to absorb liquid and expand in the stomach can help curb appetite and promote weight loss. Furthermore, when combined with a balanced diet and regular exercise, chia seeds may support weightloss goals effectively.

Bone Health

The combination of calcium, magnesium, and phosphorus found in chia seeds contributes to maintaining strong bones and teeth. These minerals are crucial for bone density and overall skeletal health, making chiaseeds an excellent dietary choice for those seeking to bolster their bone health.

Blood Sugar Regulation

The fiber and protein content in chia seeds can help regulate blood sugar levels. By slowing down the absorption of sugar in the bloodstream, chia seeds can prevent spikes in blood glucose, making them a smart choice for individuals managing diabetes or blood sugar concerns.

Culinary Versatility

One of the most appealing aspects of chia seeds is their versatility in cooking and baking. They can be easily incorporated into a variety of dishes, from smoothies and yogurt to baked goods and salads. Here are some popular ways to enjoy chia seeds:

Chia Pudding: Mix chia seeds with your choice of milk (dairy or plant-based), sweeten with honey or maple syrup, and let it sit in the refrigerator overnight. In the morning, you'll have a delicious, nutritious pudding that can be topped with fruits, nuts, or granola.

Smoothies: Toss a tablespoon of chia seeds into your favorite smoothie for an added boost of nutrition and a pleasant texture.

Baking: Substitute eggs with chia seed gel (1 tablespoon of chia seeds mixed with 3 tablespoons of water) in recipes for baked goods like muffins, pancakes, or bread.

Salads: Sprinkle chia seeds over salads for added crunch and nutrition, or mix them into salad dressings for a nutritious kick.

Energy Bars: Incorporate chia seeds into homemade energy bars or granola for a healthy snack on the go.

Nutritional Profile of Chia Seeds

This chapter delves into the nutritional composition of chia seeds, explores the health benefits associated with their consumption, and examines how they can be effectively incorporated into our diets.

Nutritional Composition### Macronutrients
Chia seeds are often touted for their unique balance of macronutrients, making them an excellent addition to a healthy diet. A typical serving size of 28 grams (about 2 tablespoons) of chia seeds provides the following:

Calories: Approximately 138 kcal
Protein: 4.7 grams

Carbohydrates: 12 grams
Fat: 8.6 grams
Saturated Fat: 0.9 grams
Monounsaturated Fat: 0.5 grams
Polyunsaturated Fat: 6.3 grams, including omega-3 and omega-6 fatty acids

Chia seeds are predominantly composed of healthy fats, particularly omega-3 fatty acids in the form of alpha-linolenic acid (ALA). The high fiber content, making up about 10.6 grams per serving, contributes to its status as a filling and satiating food.

Micronutrients

In addition to the macronutrients, chia seeds are packed with essential vitamins and minerals. Key micronutrients include:

Calcium: 177 mg (about 18% of the daily value)
Iron: 2.2 mg (about 12% of the daily value)
Magnesium: 95 mg (about 24% of the daily value)
Phosphorus: 265 mg (about 27% of the daily value)
Zinc: 1.0 mg (about 7% of the daily value)
Manganese: 0.6 mg (about 30% of the daily value)

Additionally, chia seeds are a source of antioxidants, such as flavonoids, which help combat oxidative stress and may lower the risk of chronic diseases.

Fiber Content

The noteworthy fiber content of chia seeds deserves

special emphasis. The majority of the carbohydrates in chia seeds are dietary fiber, which can be categorized into soluble and insoluble fibers.

Soluble Fiber: Forms a gel-like consistency when mixed with water, which slows down digestion and promotes a feeling of fullness, aiding in weight management.
Insoluble Fiber: Adds bulk to stool and helps maintain healthy bowel movements, reducing the risk of constipation.

This dual fiber composition supports digestive health, stabilizes blood sugar levels, and promotes hearthealth by helping lower cholesterol.

Health Benefits### Heart Health

The omega-3 fatty acids found in chia seeds play a significant role in promoting cardiovascular health. Regular consumption can reduce inflammation, improve cholesterol levels, and regulate blood pressure. The high fiber content can also contribute to lowering cholesterol levels, further protecting heart health.

Bone Health

Chia seeds are an excellent source of calcium, magnesium, phosphorus, and protein, all of which are vital for maintaining strong bones. Their nutrient profile makes them a valuable addition to plant-based diets that may lack these minerals.

Weight Management

Chia seeds can be beneficial for weight management due to their high fiber and protein content, which help promote satiety and reduce overall calorie intake. When hydrating, chia seeds absorb significant water, expanding in size and contributing to a feeling of fullness.

Blood Sugar Regulation

The soluble fiber present in chia seeds may help to slow the absorption of sugars into the bloodstream, leading to a more stable blood sugar level. This characteristic makes them suitable for individuals with diabetes or those looking to manage their glucose levels.

Digestive Health

The high fiber content in chia seeds promotes a healthy digestive system by supporting regular bowel movements and preventing constipation. Additionally, the gel-forming properties of soluble fiber can aid in maintaining a healthy gut environment.

Incorporating Chia Seeds into Your Diet

Chia seeds can be easily added to a variety of meals and snacks. Here are some ideas for incorporating them into your diet:

Smoothies: Blend chia seeds into your favorite smoothie recipes for an added nutritional boost.

Oatmeal and Yogurt: Stir chia seeds into oatmeal or yogurt for added texture and nutrition.

Baking: Use chia seeds as an ingredient in baked goods, such as muffins, bread, or pancakes.

Salads: Sprinkle chia seeds over salads or incorporate them into salad dressings for a crunchyaddition.

Puddings: Combine chia seeds with milk or a milk alternative to create a nutritious chia pudding, flavored with fruit or spices.

In summary, chia seeds stand out as a nutrient-dense food offering a plethora of health benefits. Their uniqueblend of macronutrients and micronutrients makes them a functional food, ideally suited for enhancing overall health and wellness.

How Chia Seeds Aid Digestion

One particular superfood that has gained significant attention for its myriad health benefits is the humble chia seed. Small in size but packed with nutrients, these tiny seeds are not just a culinary trend; they are a powerful ally in promoting healthy digestion. In this chapter, we will explore how chia seeds can support digestive health, the mechanisms behind their benefits, and practical ways to incorporate them into your diet.

The Nutritional Profile of Chia Seeds

Chia seeds, derived from the Salvia hispanica plant native to Central America, have been consumed for centuries by ancient civilizations. Just a tablespoon of these nutrient-rich seeds contains impressive amounts of fiber, protein, omega-3 fatty acids, and essential minerals such as calcium, magnesium, and phosphorus. However, it's the high fiber content that plays a crucial role in enhancing digestive health.

Fiber: The Digestive Champion

Fiber is a type of carbohydrate that the body cannot digest. It passes through the digestive tract largely intact, which is essential for digestive health. Chia seeds are particularly high in soluble fiber, which absorbs water and forms a gel-like substance in the stomach. This characteristic not only aids in boosting satiety, helping to control appetite, but also supports digestive well-being in several key ways:

Promoting Healthy Bowel Movements: The gel-like consistency formed when chia seeds are mixed with liquid helps soften stool and makes it easier to pass through the intestines. This can prevent constipation and promote regular bowel movements.

Feeding Beneficial Gut Bacteria: The soluble fiber in chia seeds acts as a prebiotic, providing nourishment for the beneficial bacteria residing in the gut. A healthy microbiome is vital for optimal digestion and overall health, as these bacteria play a role in breaking down food and synthesizing essential nutrients.

Controlling Blood Sugar Levels: Chia seeds can slow the absorption of glucose in the bloodstream,which helps prevent spikes in blood sugar levels. This regulation is particularly beneficial for those with digestive concerns related to diabetes, as it supports a more stable digestive process.

Hydration and Detoxification

Another remarkable feature of chia seeds is their ability to absorb water—up to 12 times their weight. When consumed, they expand in the stomach, which can lead to a feeling of fullness and help individuals consciously regulate their food intake. The influx of water from chia seeds can also assist in keeping the digestive system hydrated, promoting efficient digestion and helping to flush waste from the body.

Moreover, chia seeds can aid in detoxification. As they traverse the digestive tract, they help bind to toxinsand waste products, promoting their elimination from the body. This detoxifying effect can reduce the burden on the liver and enhance overall digestive function.

Incorporating Chia Seeds into Your Diet

Given their numerous health benefits, incorporating chia seeds into your diet is both easy and enjoyable. Here are some practical tips on how to include them in your daily meals:

Chia Pudding: A popular and versatile option is chia

pudding. Combine chia seeds with your choice of milk (dairy or plant-based), sweeten with honey or maple syrup, and let it sit overnight in the refrigerator. In the morning, top with fruits, nuts, or granola for a nutritious breakfast.

Smoothies: Add a tablespoon of chia seeds to your smoothies to boost the fiber and nutrient content. They can complement a variety of flavors without altering the taste.

Baking: Chia seeds can be incorporated into baked goods, such as muffins, bread, or cookies. They not only enhance the nutritional value but also add a delightful crunch.

Salads and Soups: Sprinkle chia seeds on salads, soups, or even yogurt to enhance texture and nutrition. Their neutral flavor makes them a versatile addition to both savory and sweet dishes.

Hydration: Mix chia seeds with water or your favorite beverage and let them soak for a few minutes. This can create a hydrating drink that is both refreshing and beneficial for digestion.

Chia seeds are a nutritional powerhouse that can significantly aid digestion through their high fiber content, hydration properties, and detoxification benefits. By embracing these tiny seeds, you can empower your digestive health, improve regularity, and support your overall well-being.

Chapter 3: Preparing for the Cleanse of the body with chia seeds

In this chapter, we'll delve into the remarkable potential of chia seeds as a nutrient-dense companion for body cleansing, while also exploring how to prepare ourselves—physically, emotionally, and mentally—for this transformative health journey.

The Power of Chia Seeds

Chia seeds, sourced from the *Salvia hispanica* plant native to Central America, have been cherished for centuries by the Aztecs and Mayans, not only as a source of energy but also for their extensive health benefits.

When soaked in water or other liquids, these small seeds swell up and create a gel-like substance that aids digestion, boosts hydration, and fosters a sense of fullness. Packed with omega-3 fatty acids, fiber, protein, and vital minerals, chia seeds are an excellent way to support your body throughout the cleansing process.

Before you begin your cleanse, it's important to grasp what it means to detoxify your body. A cleanse can help eliminate toxins, decrease inflammation, promote gut health, and strengthen your immune system. By integrating chia seeds into your cleanse, you prepare both your body and mind for a meaningful journey toward improved well-being.

Mental Preparation: Setting Intentions

Cleansing involves as much mental preparation as it does physical readiness. Take some time to reflect on your motivations for wanting to cleanse your body. Are you aiming for more energy? Do you wish to enhance your digestive health? Are you looking to alleviate symptoms of inflammation or other discomforts? Document these intentions and keep them in a visible place to serve as motivation during your cleansing journey.

Incorporating mindfulness practices can be helpful at this stage. Engaging in meditation or yoga can enhance your awareness and foster a deeper connection with your body. These activities can promote relaxation, focus, and clarity, enabling you to navigate the changes ahead with confidence and positivity.

Physical Preparation: Nourishing Your Body

To ensure your body functions optimally during the cleanse, it's crucial to nourish it in the days leading up to your start date. Begin by gradually removing processed foods, refined sugars, and unhealthy fats from your diet.

Instead, prioritize whole, nutrient-rich foods such as fruits, vegetables, whole grains, nuts, and seeds. This transitional period is vital for preparing your digestive system for the higher intake of fiber and nutrients that the cleanse will entail.

Incorporating chia seeds into your meals before you start the cleanse can help your body adapt more easily. Try adding them to smoothies, oatmeal, or salads. Their high fiber content will support healthy digestion and create a sense of fullness, helping to ease any hunger pangs during your cleanse.

Hydration: The Key to Success

Adequate hydration plays a pivotal role in any cleansing process. Water is essential for flushing out toxins and supporting the functions of every cell in your body. As you prepare for your cleanse, aim to increase your water intake throughout the day. A good rule of thumb is to drink half your body weight in ounces of water daily.

Additionally, consider infusing your water with slices of lemon or cucumber to add flavor and enhance detoxification. These infused waters not only improve hydration but also provide valuable vitamins and minerals that support overall health.

Creating a Balanced Chia Seed Cleanse Protocol

A balanced approach to using chia seeds during your cleanse will help optimize their benefits. Start by determining how you want to incorporate them into your meals. Here are some ideas:

Chia Seed Pudding: Mix chia seeds with almond milk (or any preferred milk alternative) and let it sit overnight in the refrigerator. Top with fresh fruits, nuts, or a drizzle of honey to enhance flavors.

Smoothies: Blend chia seeds with your favorite fruits, leafy greens, and a source of protein (like Greek yogurt or a protein powder). This adds texture and nutritional density to your smoothies.

Chia Seed Gel: Mix one part chia seeds with three parts water and allow it to thicken. This gel can be added to salads, baked goods, or yogurt for a nutrient boost.

Understanding the Process and Listening to Your Body

As you prepare to embark on your chia seed cleanse, remember that this journey is unique to you. Listen to your body and trust your instincts throughout the process. Pay attention to any changes in your energy levels, digestion, or mood. Keep a journal to document your experiences, reflecting on the benefits as well as any challenges you encounter.

Preparing for a cleanse with chia seeds is about more than just the food—it is a holistic approach that encompasses mental clarity, physical nourishment, and emotional readiness. By setting clear intentions, gradually altering your diet, increasing hydration, and choosing how to incorporate chia seeds meaningfully, you empower yourself for a successful cleanse.

Setting Your Goals and Expectations for Constipation Management

Constipation is more than just a physical discomfort—it can affect your overall well-being, mental health, and quality of life. For many, the journey to managing constipation may feel overwhelming with various options available, promising quick fixes and miraculous cures.

Understanding Constipation

Before diving into goal-setting, it's essential to understand what constipation is. Defined generally as having fewer than three bowel movements per week, constipation can manifest in various ways—straining during bowel movements, feeling as though your bowels are not fully emptied, or experiencing hard, dry stools. It can result from dietary choices, lifestyle habits, medical conditions, or medications. Knowing the underlyingcauses will allow you to set more informed and realistic expectations.

Identifying Your Individual Needs

Each person's experience with constipation is unique. Therefore, your goals should reflect your specificsituation. Start by asking yourself the following questions:

What symptoms are you experiencing?
- Identify whether you're dealing with infrequent bowel movements, difficulties in passing stools, discomfort, or related issues such as bloating.

How does constipation affect your daily life?
- Consider how your symptoms impact activities like work, social interactions, and emotional well-being.

Have you tried any interventions?
- Assess past efforts—what worked, what didn't, and what changes did you notice in your symptoms? ## Setting Realistic Goals
Once you have a better understanding of your experience with constipation, you can begin setting goals. Here are some practical steps to guide you:

Define Your Desired Outcomes:
Short-term Goals: These might include increasing your fiber intake to a specific amount daily or drinking a certain amount of water each day. Short-term objectives could also include tracking bowel movements to identify patterns.
Long-term Goals: These should focus on overall well-being, such as establishing a regular bowel routine or feeling comfortable discussing bowel health with your healthcare provider.

Be Specific and Measurable:
- Instead of saying, "I want to poop more regularly," specify, "I aim to have a bowel movement at least four times a week." This clarity will help you monitor progress effectively.

Incorporate Small, Achievable Steps:
- Start with small lifestyle changes, such as adding one serving of fruits or vegetables to your diet each day or committing to a short daily walk. Gradual changes are

often more sustainable and less daunting.

Plan for Potential Setbacks:
- Recognize that change can be challenging. It's essential to be prepared for setbacks and understand they are a part of the process. Setting up a support system—whether that's family, friends, or healthcare professionals—can help you navigate these challenges.

Adjusting Your Expectations

While it's important to remain optimistic about your goals, it's equally vital to keep your expectations grounded in reality:

Understand Timeframes:
- Many changes, especially in dietary and lifestyle habits, may take time to yield results. Setting a timeline for your goals can help manage expectations; however, be flexible as your body may take longer to adjust.

Embrace Progress, Not Perfection:
- Focus on improvement rather than achieving perfection. Celebrate small victories in your journey, such as consistently drinking more water or incorporating fiber into your meals.

Consult with Professionals:
- Engage with healthcare providers, dietitians, or nutritionists for tailored advice that respects your individual health needs. They can help provide guidance on attainable goals based on your specific circumstances.

Managing constipation is a personal journey that requires you to be proactive in setting your own goals and expectations. By understanding your body, defining realistic, measurable targets, and adjusting your expectations, you can create a manageable plan that promotes both physical comfort and emotional well-being.

Essential Ingredients for Using Chia Seeds to Combat Constipation

Renowned for their impressive nutritional profile and gastrointestinal benefits, chia seeds can play a crucial role in promoting regularity and overall digestive health. In this chapter, we will explore the essential ingredients that enhance the effectiveness of chia seeds in combating constipation and discover practical ways to incorporate them into your daily routine.

The Power of Chia Seeds

Chia seeds, derived from the Salvia hispanica plant, have been utilized for centuries due to their impressive health benefits. They are rich in dietary fiber, omega-3 fatty acids, protein, and various essential vitamins and minerals. One of the standout features of chia seeds is their ability to absorb water and swell up to ten times their weight, forming a gel-like substance. This unique property can aid in softening stool and facilitating its passage through the digestive tract.

Nutritional Composition of Chia Seeds

Before delving into the essential ingredients that boost the effectiveness of chia seeds, it's vital to understand their nutritional value:

Dietary Fiber: Chia seeds contain approximately 10 grams of fiber per ounce (about 28 grams), making them an excellent source of both soluble and insoluble fiber. Soluble fiber assists in absorbing water and forming gel-like textures, while insoluble fiber adds bulk to stool.

Omega-3 Fatty Acids: These essential fatty acids help reduce inflammation in the gut and support overall health.

Proteins and Minerals: Chia seeds are a source of high-quality plant-based protein, magnesium, and calcium, which contribute to overall wellness.

With this foundational knowledge, let's explore the essential ingredients that can enhance the benefits of chia seeds for alleviating constipation.

Essential Ingredients ### 1. Hydration
One of the most critical elements for combating constipation is maintaining proper hydration. Chia seeds absorb a substantial amount of water, and combined with an adequate intake of fluids, they can prevent dehydration and soften stool.

Practical Tips:
Soak Chia Seeds: Before consumption, soak chia seeds in water, coconut water, or herbal tea for at least 30 minutes. This allows them to expand and creates a gel-like

texture that is easier to digest.
Increase Fluid Intake: Aim to drink at least eight glasses of water daily. Herbal teas, particularly those containing ginger, peppermint, or chamomile, can also provide soothing benefits to the digestive system.

2. Complementary High-Fiber Foods

Pairing chia seeds with other high-fiber foods can significantly enhance their effectiveness. Foods rich in both soluble and insoluble fiber stimulate bowel movements and support gut health.

Suggested Foods:
Fruits: Apples, pears, berries, and bananas are excellent sources of fiber. Try adding chopped fruits to your chia seed pudding or smoothies.
Vegetables: Leafy greens, carrots, and broccoli provide additional fiber. Incorporate them into salads, stir-fries, or even smoothies for a nutrient boost.
Whole Grains: Quinoa, brown rice, and oats complement chia seeds well, providing both fiber and a spectrum of nutrients.

3. Probiotics

Probiotic-rich foods can enhance digestion and overall gut health. The friendly bacteria in these foods help maintain a healthy balance in the gut microbiome, which can aid in regular bowel movements when combined with chia seeds.

Probiotic Foods to Consider:

Yogurt: Look for plain yogurt with live cultures. You can create a delicious chia seed yogurt parfait layered with fruits and nuts.
Kefir: This tangy beverage is rich in probiotics and can be mixed with chia seeds for a nutritious drink.
Fermented Vegetables: Foods like sauerkraut and kimchi not only provide probiotics but also add flavor and nutrients to your meals.

4. Healthy Fats

Incorporating healthy fats into your diet can also help promote regularity. Fats can lubricate the intestines, making stool easier to pass.

Healthy Fat Sources:
Avocado: This creamy fruit is rich in healthy fats and fiber. Add slices of avocado to salads or blend it into smoothies.
Nuts and Seeds: Almonds, walnuts, and sunflower seeds can enhance the fiber content of your meals. Use them as toppings on chia pudding or yogurt.
Olive Oil: A drizzle of extra virgin olive oil on salads or cooked vegetables can provide healthy fats, aiding in smoother digestion.

5. Liquid Additives

Certain liquids can enhance the effects of chia seeds. Adding them to various beverages can promote hydration and make it easier to consume chia regularly.

Recommended Liquids:

Coconut Water: Packed with electrolytes and a light sweetness, coconut water can add flavor to chia seed drinks.
Fruit Juices: Freshly squeezed juices, particularly those from citrus fruits, can add a refreshing twist to your chia seed concoctions while providing vitamin C.
Milk Alternatives: Almond milk, oat milk, or coconut milk can be combined with chia seeds for a creamy treat.

Incorporating chia seeds into your diet can be a game-changer for combating constipation, especially when combined with other essential ingredients. By focusing on hydration, high-fiber foods, probiotics, healthy fats, and flavorful liquids, you can create a holistic approach to digestive health.

Chapter 4: Week 1 - Starting the Journey
using chia seeds

As we embark on this week-long journey of nutritional enhancement, we'll shine a spotlight on a tiny powerhouse in the superfood realm: chia seeds. Despite their small size, chia seeds boast an impressive nutritional profile, making them an accessible and versatile choice for anyone looking to improve their diet, boost energy, or enhance overall wellness.

Day 1: Unveiling Chia Seeds

Our adventure begins with an introduction to chia seeds. These small black or white seeds, sourced from the *Salvia hispanica* plant, have gained popularity due to their remarkable health benefits. Rich in fiber, protein, omega-3 fatty acids, and various micronutrients, chia seeds can absorb up to twelve times their weight in water, creating a gel-like consistency that promotes hydration and fullness.

As you start to include chia seeds in your diet, take a moment to reflect on their fascinating history. Ancient Aztecs and Mayans cherished chia seeds for their energy-boosting properties, consuming them during long travels or battles. Today, we can tap into that same energy in our daily lives.

Day 2: Exploring Chia Seed Versatility

On day two, let's dive into the many ways to incorporate chia seeds into your meals. The true beauty of chia lies in its adaptability; it can be sprinkled over salads, blended into smoothies, or used as a thickening agent in soups and sauces.

Try making a simple *Chia Seed Pudding.* Combine three tablespoons of chia seeds with one cup of your favorite milk (dairy or plant-based). Add a sweetener like honey or maple syrup and a splash of vanilla extract. Stir the mixture well and let it sit in the refrigerator overnight. By morning, you'll have a creamy, nutritious treat ready for breakfast or a snack.

Day 3: Chia and Hydration

As we reach the midpoint of our week, let's focus on hydration—a vital yet often overlooked aspect of health. Chia seeds can significantly aid in maintaining proper hydration, thanks to their impressive water-absorbing capacity. Just one tablespoon of chia seeds can soak up up to two and a half tablespoons of liquid, helping you stay full and hydrated.

Create a refreshing *Chia Seed Lemonade* by mixing water, fresh lemon juice, and a touch of honey or agave syrup with a tablespoon of chia seeds. Allow the mixture to sit for about ten minutes, enabling the chia seeds to swell before enjoying. This delicious drink not only keeps you hydrated but also provides a boost of omega-3s and fiber for your body.

Day 4: The Nutritional Benefits

As we settle into the week, let's dive deeper into the myriad of benefits chia seeds offer. The high fiber content (approximately 10 grams per ounce) plays a crucial role in digestive health, promoting regularity and preventing constipation. Additionally, the omega-3 fatty acids found in chia seeds can support heart health by reducing inflammation and improving cholesterol levels.

To harness these benefits, consider adding chia seeds to your afternoon snack routine. A simple sprinkle over yogurt or a handful of chia seeds blended into your favorite smoothie can make a significant difference in both taste and nutrition.

Day 5: Mindful Eating with Chia

As the week progresses, it's important to incorporate mindfulness into our eating practices. Consider each meal an opportunity to reflect on your food choices and their effects on your body. Chia seeds encourage this kind of conscious eating—when incorporated thoughtfully into your diet, they can transform a simple meal into a nourishing experience.

Try taking a few moments before each meal to acknowledge the effort and intention behind your food choices. Imagine the journey of those seeds from soil to plate, and feel gratitude for the nutrition they provide.

Day 6: Experimenting with Recipes

The weekend is an excellent time for culinary exploration. It's your chance to experiment with creative recipes that showcase chia seeds. Consider whipping up a batch of *Chia Seed Jam* by simmering your favorite fruits with a bit of water and sweetener. Once the mixture cools, stir in chia seeds and let it thicken in the fridge. You can use this jam as a spread on toast, a topping for pancakes, or even as a filling in desserts.

Another great dish to try is *Chia Seed Energy Balls*. Combine chia seeds with oats, nut butter, honey, and chocolate chips. Roll them into bite-sized balls and store them in the refrigerator for a quick, nutritious energy boost throughout your busy week.

Day 7: Reflecting on Your Journey

As the first week of your journey comes to an end, take time to reflect on your experiences and the changes you've made. How do you feel physically and mentally? Are you noticing any differences in your energy levels or digestion?

This week, you've not only embraced the health benefits of chia seeds but also nurtured a relationship with your food. Remember, transformation is as much about the process as it is about the destination.
Continuously incorporating chia seeds into your diet can be a rewarding practice—a small but impactful step towards a healthier lifestyle.

Daily Meal Plans and Recipes with Chia Seeds for Constipation

While there are various remedies available, incorporating fiber-rich foods into your diet can be an effective way to promote regularity. Chia seeds, known for their high fiber content and nutritional benefits, are an excellent addition to combat constipation. This chapter will explore daily meal plans designed specifically for alleviating constipation, featuring delicious recipes that highlight the versatility of chia seeds.

Benefits of Chia Seeds

Chia seeds are tiny black seeds derived from the Salvia hispanica plant, native to Mexico and Guatemala. These superfoods are packed with nutrients, offering a wealth of health benefits:

High Fiber Content: Just one ounce (about 28 grams) of chia seeds contains approximately 11 grams of fiber, contributing to smoother digestion and regular bowel movements.

Hydration: Chia seeds can absorb up to 12 times their weight in water, helping to keep the digestive system hydrated and supporting stool softening.

Nutrient Dense: In addition to fiber, chia seeds are rich in omega-3 fatty acids, protein, antioxidants, and various vitamins and minerals.
Prebiotic Properties: They can act as prebiotics, promoting the growth of beneficial gut bacteria, which further aids digestion.

Daily Meal Plan Overview

Incorporating chia seeds into your daily diet does not have to be complicated or boring. Below is a simple daily meal plan featuring chia seed recipes designed to support digestive health and alleviate constipation. Each meal is crafted to ensure variety, taste, and nutrition.

Sample Daily Meal Plan

Breakfast: Chia Seed Pudding with Berries

Ingredients:
¼ cup chia seeds
1 cup almond milk (or any milk of choice)
1 tablespoon maple syrup (optional)
½ teaspoon vanilla extract
Fresh berries (strawberries, blueberries, raspberries)

Instructions:
In a bowl or jar, combine chia seeds, almond milk, maple syrup, and vanilla extract. Stir well to avoid clumps.
Let sit for 10 minutes, then stir again. Cover and refrigerate for at least 2 hours, or overnight.
Before serving, top with fresh berries. Enjoy chilled!

Morning Snack: Chia Seed Smoothie

Ingredients:
1 banana
1 cup spinach

1 tablespoon chia seeds
1 cup almond milk or coconut water
A handful of ice

Instructions:
Combine all ingredients in a blender and blend until smooth.
Pour into a glass and sip away, enjoying the refreshing

taste and digestive benefits!

Lunch: Quinoa Salad with Chia Vinaigrette

Ingredients:
1 cup cooked quinoa
½ cup cherry tomatoes, halved
½ cucumber, diced
¼ cup red onion, finely chopped
¼ cup olives
Fresh parsley for garnish
Chia Vinaigrette:
2 tablespoons chia seeds
3 tablespoons olive oil
2 tablespoons apple cider vinegar
Salt and pepper to taste

Instructions:
To prepare the vinaigrette, whisk together chia seeds, olive oil, apple cider vinegar, salt, and pepper in a small bowl. Let it sit for 10-15 minutes to thicken slightly.
In a large bowl, mix cooked quinoa, tomatoes, cucumber, red onion, and olives. Drizzle with the chiavinaigrette and toss gently to combine.
Garnish with fresh parsley and enjoy a refreshing, fiber-rich lunch.

Afternoon Snack: Chia Seed and Nut Energy Balls

Ingredients:
1 cup dates, pitted
½ cup almonds or walnuts
2 tablespoons chia seeds

1 tablespoon cocoa powder (optional)
A pinch of salt
Unsweetened coconut flakes (optional)

Instructions:
In a food processor, blend dates and nuts until finely chopped.
Add chia seeds, cocoa powder (if using), and salt. Pulse until the mixture is thick and sticky.
Roll the mixture into small balls and coat with coconut flakes if desired. Refrigerate for a firm texture.

Dinner: Grilled Veggies and Chia Seed Pasta

Ingredients:
2 cups mixed vegetables (zucchini, bell peppers, mushrooms)
1 tablespoon olive oil
Salt and pepper to taste
½ cup cooked whole grain pasta
1 tablespoon chia seeds
Fresh basil for garnish

Instructions:
Preheat a grill or grill pan over medium heat.
Toss vegetables with olive oil, salt, and pepper. Grill for 6-8 minutes or until tender.
In a bowl, mix grilled veggies with cooked pasta and chia seeds. Toss well.
Garnish with fresh basil before serving.

Evening Treat: Chia Seed Popsicles

Ingredients:
1 cup coconut water or fruit juice
2 tablespoons chia seeds
Fresh fruits (optional)

Instructions:
In a bowl, combine coconut water or juice with chia seeds.
Stir well.
Allow to sit for about 10 minutes, then stir again.
Pour the mixture into popsicle molds, adding pieces of fresh fruit if desired.
Freeze for at least 4 hours before enjoying a refreshing treat!

Integrating chia seeds into your daily meals can be an effective and delicious way to enhance your fiber intake and support digestive health. The meal plan and recipes provided in this chapter not only focus on alleviating constipation but also highlight the versatility and nutritional benefits of chia seeds.

Defining the best times to use chia seeds to controlconstipation

Packed with fiber, omega-3 fatty acids, antioxidants, and essential minerals, chia seeds are particularly noteworthy for their role in promoting digestive health. This chapter aims to explore the optimal times toincorporate chia seeds into your diet for effective constipation relief.

Understanding Chia Seeds and Their Benefits for Digestion

Before delving into timing, it's essential to understand why chia seeds are beneficial for those struggling with constipation. Chia seeds are remarkably high in soluble fiber, which absorbs water and forms a gel-like substance during digestion. This process not only aids in nutrient absorption but also helps to soften and bulk up stool, making it easier to pass.

The Fiber Factor

In just two tablespoons (approx. 28 grams) of chia seeds, you can find about 11 grams of dietary fiber. This substantial fiber content can promote regular bowel movements and improve overall gut health. However, timing your consumption effectively is crucial in maximizing these benefits.

Best Times to Consume Chia Seeds### 1. **Morning Kickstart**
One of the best times to incorporate chia seeds into your diet is during breakfast. Soaking chia seeds overnight in water, almond milk, or yogurt transforms them into a pudding-like texture that is not only delicious but also easy for your body to digest. Consuming chia pudding or a smoothie with chia seeds in the morning can help jumpstart your metabolism and encourage bowel movements throughout the day.

Example Recipe: Chia Seed Breakfast Pudding

Ingredients:
2 tablespoons chia seeds

1 cup of unsweetened almond milk
1 teaspoon honey or maple syrup (optional)
Fresh fruits (berries, banana slices, etc.)

Instructions:
Mix chia seeds with almond milk, sweetener, and any additional flavors.
Stir well and let sit overnight in the refrigerator.
Top with fruits before serving in the morning.### 2. **As a Pre-Meal Supplement**
Incorporating chia seeds into your pre-meal routine can also boost your digestive health. Consuming them about 30 minutes before meals can promote a feeling of fullness, helping to prevent overeating. Additionally, this allows the seeds to absorb some water and swell, preparing your digestive system for the upcoming meal, which can help in forming softer stools.

3. **Hydration at Critical Moments**

Chia seeds in water can be particularly beneficial when experiencing the initial signs of constipation. When mixed in water, they hydrate quickly and expand. Drinking a glass of chia seed water can be a game-changer in stimulating bowel movements. This is particularly beneficial if you find yourself feeling bloated or constipated after a long period of inactivity, such as during travel or prolonged sitting at work.

Chia Seed Water Recipe

Ingredients:
1 tablespoon chia seeds

1 cup water
A squeeze of lemon (optional)

Instructions:
Soak chia seeds in water for about 15-30 minutes until they swell.
Add lemon for flavor and drink promptly. ### 4. **Evening Relaxation**
Finally, incorporating chia seeds into your evening routine can also aid digestion. A soothing evening smoothie or yogurt bowl with chia seeds can not only help settle your stomach but also prepare your body for digestion overnight. Consuming fiber-rich foods in the evening ensures that your digestive system is equipped to process waste efficiently.

Considerations and Guidelines

While chia seeds are an excellent addition to your diet, moderation is key. Overconsumption of fiber can lead to bloating and discomfort, particularly if your body isn't accustomed to increased fiber intake. It's advisable to start with one to two tablespoons per day and gradually increase your intake as your digestive system adapts.

Staying Hydrated

Chia seeds absorb a significant amount of water, so it is crucial to drink plenty of fluids throughout the day when consuming them. Hydration is vital in ensuring that fiber can do its job of softening and bulking up stool effectively.

Incorporating chia seeds into your diet can significantly

enhance digestion and alleviate constipation when consumed strategically. By understanding the best times—whether at breakfast, before meals, as a response to early signs of constipation, or in the evening—you can optimize the benefits of these tiny powerhouses.

Chapter 5: Week 2 - Deepening the Cleanse of the body with Chia seeds

These tiny yet powerful seeds offer remarkable benefits, making them the perfect ally in our pursuit of optimal health. In this chapter, we will explore how to integrate chia seeds into our diet, their nutritional profile, and the countless ways they can enhance our body's natural detoxification processes.

Understanding Chia Seeds

Chia seeds come from the *Salvia hispanica* plant, native to Mexico and Guatemala. These small black and white seeds are renowned for their impressive nutritional content. A rich source of fiber, omega-3 fatty acids, antioxidants, and essential minerals like calcium, magnesium, and phosphorus, chia seeds can significantly contribute to your overall well-being.

Nutritional Breakdown

Fiber: Chia seeds are reputed to be one of the highest plant-based sources of fiber. Each ounce (approximately 28 grams) contains about 10 grams of fiber, promoting healthy digestion, satiety, and regulating blood sugar levels.

Omega-3 Fatty Acids: Chia seeds are a plant-based source of alpha-linolenic acid (ALA), making them an excellent choice for those looking to increase their omega-3 intake. This fatty acid is known for its anti-inflammatory properties and its role in promoting heart health.

Protein: While not a complete protein, chia seeds provide all nine essential amino acids, making them a great addition to vegetarian and vegan diets. **Antioxidants:** Packed with antioxidants, chia seeds help combat oxidative stress in the body, which can lead to chronic diseases.

Benefits of Chia Seeds in Detoxification

In our quest for cleansing, chia seeds offer several benefits that can support the body's detoxification process:

Hydration: When soaked in water, chia seeds expand and form a gel-like consistency. This property not only helps retain moisture in the digestive tract but also supports proper hydration, which is crucial during a cleanse.

Digestive Relief: The soluble fiber in chia seeds acts like a sponge, absorbing water and forming a gel that can help soothe inflammation in the digestive tract. This is especially beneficial during detoxification, as a well-functioning digestive system is essential for effective cleansing.

Detoxifying Properties: Chia seeds are abundant in fiber, which helps bind to toxins and waste products in our digestive system, facilitating their elimination from the body. This promotes regular bowel movements and enhances liver function, both vital aspects of detoxification.

Blood Sugar Regulation: The fiber and healthy fats in chia seeds can help stabilize blood sugar levels, reducing cravings and providing sustained energy. This stability is beneficial during a cleanse, as it helps mitigate potential energy dips.

Incorporating Chia Seeds into the Diet

Integrating chia seeds into your meals can be seamless and enjoyable. Here are some delicious ways to incorporate them into your day:

1. Chia Seed Pudding

Chia seed pudding is a flavorful and nutritious option for breakfast or a snack. To prepare, combine ¼ cup of chia seeds with 1 cup of your choice of milk (dairy, almond, coconut, etc.) and sweeten with honey or maple syrup. Let the mixture sit in the refrigerator overnight. In the morning, add fresh fruit, nuts, or seeds for added texture and flavor.

2. Smoothies

Add a tablespoon of chia seeds to your morning smoothie. They blend seamlessly into any mix of fruits and vegetables, adding a nutritional boost without altering the taste. Try pairing them with spinach, banana, and almond milk for a refreshing detox smoothie.

3. Salads and Dressings

Sprinkle chia seeds over salads or mix them into homemade salad dressings for extra crunch and nutrition. Their mild flavor won't interfere with the dish, yet they offer a satisfying texture.

4. Baking

Substitute a portion of flour in your baking recipes, such as muffins or pancakes, with chia seeds. Alternatively, create a chia egg by mixing 1 tablespoon of chia seeds with 2.5 tablespoons of water, letting it sit until it becomes gel-like. This can replace one egg in vegan recipes.

5. Soups and Stews

Chia seeds can also be added to soups and stews as a thickening agent. Simply stir in a tablespoon or two while the dish simmers, which will not only enhance texture but also boost its nutritional profile.

As we navigate through Week 2 of our detox journey, chia seeds serve as a crucial component in deepening our cleanse. By integrating these nutrient-dense seeds into our diet, we're not only supporting our body's natural detoxification processes but also providing it with essential nutrients.

Practical and effective recipes with Chia seeds for constipation

When dietary choices fall short, incorporating certain superfoods like chia seeds into your meals can be a game-changer. Not only are chia seeds packed with nutrients, but they are also high in fiber and can help promote regular bowel movements. In this chapter, we will explore a variety of practical and effective recipes that leverage the unique properties of chia seeds to alleviate constipation and promote digestive health.

Understanding the Benefits of Chia Seeds

Chia seeds are tiny black seeds derived from the Salvia hispanica plant, native to Mexico and Guatemala. They are a powerhouse of nutrients, offering:

High Fiber Content: Chia seeds contain about 11 grams of fiber per ounce, which can help support healthy digestion and regularity.

Hydrophilic Properties: When soaked in liquid, chia seeds can absorb up to 12 times their weight in water, forming a gel-like consistency. This property can help bulk up stool and facilitate easier passage through the digestive tract.

Omega-3 Fatty Acids: Chia seeds are an excellent source of plant-based omega-3 fatty acids, which are important for overall health.

Rich in Antioxidants: These seeds contain antioxidants that help combat oxidative stress in the body.

By incorporating chia seeds into your diet, you can significantly improve your digestive health. Below are several easy and delicious recipes that utilize chia seeds to combat constipation effectively.

1. Chia Seed Pudding### Ingredients:
1/4 cup chia seeds

1 cup almond milk (or any milk of choice)
1 tablespoon maple syrup or honey (optional)
1/2 teaspoon vanilla extract
Fresh fruit (such as berries or banana) for topping

Instructions:
In a mixing bowl, combine chia seeds, almond milk, maple syrup, and vanilla extract. Stir well to ensure there are no clumps of chia seeds.
Let the mixture sit for about 10 minutes, then stir again to break up any clumps that may have formed.
Cover the bowl and refrigerate for at least 2 hours or overnight.
When ready to serve, give the pudding a good stir and top it with fresh fruit. Enjoy it as a nutritious breakfast or a satisfying snack!
2. Chia Seed Smoothie ### Ingredients:
1 tablespoon chia seeds
1 banana
1/2 cup spinach (optional)

1 cup unsweetened almond milk (or any milk of choice)
1 tablespoon peanut butter (optional)
Ice cubes (optional)

Instructions:
Place all ingredients in a blender.
Blend until smooth, adding ice cubes if desired for a chilled effect.
Pour into a glass and enjoy the creamy, nutrient-dense smoothie. This recipe packs a fiber punch that can help promote bowel regularity.
3. Chia Seed Jam ### Ingredients:
2 cups mixed berries (fresh or frozen)
2 tablespoons chia seeds
1-2 tablespoons honey or maple syrup (to taste)
1 tablespoon lemon juice

Instructions:
In a saucepan over medium heat, combine the berries and lemon juice. Cook until the berries are soft and starting to break down, about 5-7 minutes.
Remove the saucepan from heat and stir in the honey or maple syrup.
Mash the mixture slightly with a fork or potato masher.
Stir in the chia seeds and mix well. Let the mixture sit for about 10-15 minutes to thicken up.
Store in a jar in the refrigerator for up to a week. Spread this delicious jam on whole-grain toast or mix it into yogurt for a fiber-rich treat.
4. Chia Seed Energy Bites ### Ingredients:
1 cup rolled oats
1/2 cup nut butter (peanut, almond, or cashew)
1/4 cup honey or maple syrup

1/4 cup chia seeds
1/4 cup dark chocolate chips (optional)
1/4 cup shredded coconut (optional)

Instructions:
In a large mixing bowl, combine all ingredients and mix thoroughly until well combined.
Using your hands, form the mixture into small balls, about the size of a tablespoon.
Place the energy bites on a baking sheet lined with parchment paper and refrigerate for about 30 minutesto firm up.
Store the bites in an airtight container in the fridge. Enjoy them as a convenient snack throughout theweek!

Incorporating chia seeds into your diet is a simple and delicious way to help manage constipation and promote digestive health. Whether you prefer them in a creamy pudding, a refreshing smoothie, a sweet jam, or convenient energy bites, chia seeds can easily be added to your daily meals.

Dealing with Detox Symptoms with Chia seeds

People turn to detox diets to eliminate toxins, boost energy, enhance mental clarity, and promote overall vitality. While detoxing can yield significant benefits, it can also trigger a variety of unpleasant symptoms asthe body adjusts to changes. Here, we will explore how chia seeds can be a powerful ally in managing detox symptoms, easing the transition, and supporting your overall well-being.

Understanding Detox Symptoms

Before delving into the specifics of chia seeds, it's essential to understand what detox symptoms are. Whenembarking on a detox program—whether through dietary changes, fasting, or other methods—many people experience symptoms such as:

Fatigue
Headaches
Digestive issues (bloating, constipation, diarrhea)
Mood swings
Cravings for sugar and unhealthy foods
Skin breakouts

These reactions can occur as the body begins to eliminate accumulated toxins. While they are oftentemporary, they can feel uncomfortable and disorienting. Therefore, finding ways to mitigate these symptoms is crucial for maintaining motivation and commitment throughout the detox process.

The Nutritional Power of Chia Seeds

Chia seeds, tiny black or white seeds derived from the Salvia hispanica plant, are nutritional powerhouses.They are packed with essential nutrients, including:

Omega-3 Fatty Acids: Known for their anti-inflammatory properties, omega-3s support brain health and help mitigate mood swings during detox.
Fiber: Chia seeds are rich in soluble and insoluble fiber, which can aid digestion and alleviate bowel irregularities often associated with detoxing.
Protein: A complete source of protein, chia seeds help sustain energy levels and curb cravings.
Antioxidants: High in antioxidants, chia seeds assist the body in combating oxidative stress and support the liver in its detoxification role.

Incorporating chia seeds into your diet during a detox can help counteract the adverse symptoms you may experience.

How Chia Seeds Help Alleviate Detox Symptoms
1. Easing Digestive Discomfort
Digestive issues are among the most common detox symptoms. The high fiber content in chia seeds can promote healthy bowel movements by absorbing water and creating a gel-like substance. This not only helps with constipation but also supports overall gut health by nurturing beneficial gut bacteria.

How to Use: Mix chia seeds into smoothies, yogurt, or oatmeal, or make chia pudding to increase fiber intake without feeling bloated.

2. Boosting Energy Levels

Fatigue can accompany detoxification as your body works hard to eliminate toxins. This is where the protein and healthy fats in chia seeds can play a role. They provide sustained energy without causing spikes in blood sugar, which is particularly helpful when cravings hit.

How to Use: Blend chia seeds into energy bites or protein shakes to create a nourishing snack that supports energy levels.

3. Balancing Mood Swings

Mood swings can be prevalent during detox, often exacerbated by the elimination of sugar and other cravings. Chia seeds contain mood-enhancing nutrients, such as omega-3 fatty acids, which can positively impact brain health and emotional well-being.

How to Use: Incorporate chia seeds into dishes like granola or smoothie bowls for a mood-lifting boost.### 4. Supporting Hydration
Staying hydrated is essential during detoxification as it aids the body in flushing out toxins. Chia seeds can absorb up to 10-12 times their weight in water, helping to keep you hydrated longer. This gelatinous quality can soothe digestive discomfort as well.

How to Use: Prepare a chia seed drink by soaking the seeds in water or coconut water, adding a splash of lemon or lime for flavor.

5. Curbing Cravings

Chia seeds can help quell cravings due to their high fiber and protein content. When consumed, they expand in the stomach, creating a feeling of fullness and satisfaction. This can be especially beneficial when eliminating sugar and processed foods during detox.

How to Use: Incorporate chia seeds into your meals as a thickener or texture enhancer. Consider adding them to soups, salads, or baked goods.

Delicious Chia Seed Recipes for Detoxification ### Chia Seed Detox Smoothie
Ingredients:
1 cup spinach
1 banana
1 tablespoon chia seeds
1 cup almond milk (or any plant-based milk)
1 tablespoon almond butter (optional)
A pinch of cinnamon

Instructions:
In a blender, combine spinach, banana, almond milk, almond butter, and cinnamon.
Blend until smooth.
Add chia seeds and pulse a few times to mix. Pour into a glass and enjoy the refreshing detox twist! ### Chia Seed Pudding

Ingredients:
1/2 cup almond milk
1/4 cup chia seeds
1 tablespoon maple syrup or honey (to taste)
Fresh fruit and nuts for toppings

Instructions:

In a bowl or jar, mix almond milk, chia seeds, and maple syrup.
Stir well to combine and let sit for at least 30 minutes or overnight in the refrigerator.
Top with fresh fruit and nuts before serving.

Detoxing can be a transformative experience, but it's not always easy. Understanding that detox symptoms are a natural part of the process can help you remain patient and committed. Incorporating chia seeds into your diet offers a myriad of benefits that can effectively alleviate these symptoms.

Chapter 6: Week 3 - Maximizing Benefits with Chia Seeds

These tiny, nutrient-rich seeds are not only incredibly sustainable but also versatile and easy to incorporate into our daily meals. This chapter aims to explore the countless benefits of chia seeds, the various ways to include them in your diet, and creative recipes that will help you maximize their advantages.

Understanding Chia Seeds

Chia seeds, derived from the *Salvia hispanica* plant native to Mexico and Guatemala, have been consumed for thousands of years. Known for their rich nutritional profile, they are an excellent source of omega-3 fatty acids, fiber, protein, and a variety of essential vitamins and minerals. The name "chia" comes from the Mayan word meaning "strength," reflecting the energy-boosting properties attributed to these seeds by ancient civilizations.

Nutritional Benefits

Nutrient-Dense: Just one ounce (approximately 28 grams) of chia seeds contains 11 grams of fiber, 5 grams of protein, and a substantial dose of omega-3 fatty acids. They are also rich in calcium, magnesium, and phosphorus, promoting bone health.

High in Antioxidants: Chia seeds are an excellent source of antioxidants that help combat oxidative stress in the body, potentially reducing the risk of chronic diseases.

Hydration and Weight Control: When soaked in liquid, chia seeds can absorb up to 12 times their weight in water, forming a gel-like substance. This characteristic can help keep you hydrated and promote a feeling of fullness, aiding in weight control by curbing cravings.

Incorporating Chia Seeds into Your Diet

One of the most appealing aspects of chia seeds is their versatility. They have a mild flavor, making them easy to add to both sweet and savory dishes. Here are several ways to maximize the benefits of chia seeds in your daily meals:

Chia Pudding: A popular choice for breakfast or a snack, chia pudding requires just three ingredients: chia seeds, liquid (such as almond milk, coconut milk, or yogurt), and a sweetener (like honey or maple syrup). Combine these ingredients, let them sit for a few hours or overnight, and enjoy a nutritious snack topped with fruits, nuts, or granola.

Smoothies: Add a tablespoon of chia seeds to your daily smoothie for a nutritional boost. They enhance the texture and provide a creamy consistency without overpowering the flavor.

Baked Goods: Incorporating chia seeds into your baking routine is another fantastic way to enhance nutrition. Add them to muffins, bread, or energy bars for extra fiber and protein.

Salads and Dressings: Sprinkle raw chia seeds over salads for a delightful crunch. You can also incorporate chia into homemade dressings to enhance the nutrient profile.

Soups and Stews: Chia seeds can be used as a thickening agent in soups and stews. Simply stir in a tablespoon or two as they cook, allowing them to absorb liquid and create a heartier dish.

Creative Chia Seed Recipes

Now that we've covered how to incorporate chia seeds into your meals, let's explore some creative, easy-to-follow recipes that will make the most of these superfoods.

1. Mango Chia Pudding

Ingredients:
1 cup coconut milk
1/2 cup chia seeds
2 ripe mangoes, pureed
1 tablespoon maple syrup
A pinch of salt

Instructions:
In a bowl, whisk together coconut milk, chia seeds, maple syrup, and salt.
Cover and let it sit in the refrigerator for at least 4 hours or overnight.
Once thickened, layer the chia pudding with mango puree in serving glasses.

Top with fresh mango slices and coconut flakes, if desired.
2. Chia Seed Smoothie Bowl
Ingredients:
1 banana
1/2 cup almond milk
1 tablespoon chia seeds
1 tablespoon almond butter
Toppings: sliced fruits, nuts, granola

Instructions:
In a blender, combine banana, almond milk, chia seeds, and almond butter. Blend until smooth.
Pour into a bowl and top with your favorite sliced fruits, nuts, and granola.#### 3. Chia Seed Energy Bites
Ingredients:
1 cup oats
1/2 cup nut butter (peanut, almond, or cashew)
1/4 cup honey or maple syrup
1/4 cup chia seeds
1/2 cup dark chocolate chips or dried fruit

Instructions:
In a mixing bowl, combine oats, nut butter, honey, chia seeds, and chocolate chips.
Roll the mixture into small balls and place them on a baking sheet.
Refrigerate for 30 minutes to firm up. Store in the refrigerator for quick snacks.

As we wrap up Week 3, it's evident that chia seeds offer numerous health benefits, making them a worthy addition to our daily diet. Whether you're looking to enhance your morning smoothie, whip up a delicious pudding for dessert, or simply need a nutritious snack, chia seeds provide an easy and effective way to boost your intake of essential nutrients.

Optimizing Your Chia Seed Intake

This chapter will guide you through various aspects of incorporating chia seeds into your diet for maximum nutritional advantage.

Understanding Nutrition: What Chia Seeds Offer

Before diving into practical tips for optimization, it is essential to understand what makes chia seeds nutritionally unique. Here are some key components:

Rich in Nutrients: Chia seeds are an excellent source of essential nutrients such as calcium, magnesium, iron, and zinc. They also deliver a healthy dose of fiber, which is vital for digestive health.

High in Omega-3s: These tiny seeds are one of the best plant-based sources of omega-3 fatty acids, specifically alpha-linolenic acid (ALA), which supports heart health.

Antioxidants: Chia seeds are rich in antioxidants that combat oxidative stress and inflammation, contributing to overall wellness.

Versatile and Satiety-Enhancing: Due to their ability to absorb water and expand in the stomach, chia seeds promote a feeling of fullness and may help with weight management.

Optimal Consumption: How to Incorporate Chia Seeds
1. Daily Serving Size
Moderation is key when including chia seeds in your diet. A typical serving size is about 1 to 2 tablespoons(15 to 30 grams) per day. This amount provides substantial benefits without overwhelming your digestive system. If you're new to chia seeds, starting with one teaspoon and gradually increasing to your desired amount can help your body adjust.

2. Preparation Methods

To maximize their nutritional benefits, chia seeds can be prepared in several ways:

Soaking: Soaking chia seeds in water or milk for a few hours or overnight helps them absorb liquid and develop a gel-like consistency, making them easier to digest. This method is excellent for making chia puddings or smoothies.

Grinding: Grinding chia seeds into a powder can enhance their digestibility and nutrient absorption, especially for those who may have difficulty breaking down the tough outer shell of the seed.

Incorporation into Recipes: Chia seeds can be easily added to various recipes, including:
Smoothies: Blend chia seeds into your morning smoothie for an energy boost.

Baked Goods: Substitute chia seeds for eggs in vegan recipes or add them to muffins, breads, andpancakes.

Salads and Dressings: Sprinkle chia seeds on salads or mix them into dressings for added texture andnutrition.

Soups and Stews: Stir in chia seeds while cooking soups or stews to thicken the consistency.### 3. Timing and Pairing Timing your chia seed consumption can also play a role in optimizing their benefits. Here are some suggestions:

Breakfast Boost: Incorporate chia seeds into oatmeal or yogurt in the morning for sustained energythroughout the day.

Pre-Workout Snack: Consuming chia seeds before a workout can provide a quick source of energy and hydration, thanks to their high fiber and water-absorbing properties.

Hydration: Consider drinking chia seed water or a chia refresher—simply mix chia seeds with water and a splash of lemon juice for a hydrating drink.

Listening to Your Body

As with any dietary change, it's essential to listen to your body when incorporating chia seeds into your routine. Pay attention to how you feel after consuming them, particularly regarding digestion and energy levels. Some people might experience bloating if they consume too many chia seeds too quickly, while others may find them soothing to the digestive system. Adjust your intake based on your personal experience.

Storage and Freshness

To maintain the freshness and nutritional integrity of chia seeds, store them in a cool, dark place, preferably in an airtight container. Although chia seeds have a long shelf life, consuming them within six months after opening is ideal to enjoy their full flavor and health benefits.

Optimizing your chia seed intake can transform your health in various ways. By understanding their nutritional profile, experimenting with different preparation methods, and mindfully listening to your body, you can seamlessly incorporate these tiny but mighty seeds into your daily routine.

Incorporating Healthy Habits for Constipation Management

It isn't simply a matter of infrequent bowel movements; rather, it encompasses a range of symptoms, including straining during passage, lumpy or hard stools, a sensation of incomplete evacuation, and abdominal discomfort. To combat this condition effectively, it is crucial to adopt healthy habits that promote digestive regularity and overall well-being. This chapter delves into effective strategies and lifestyle changes, emphasizing the incorporation of healthy habits to manage and alleviate constipation.

Understanding Constipation

Before we explore the remedies, it is essential to understand the underlying causes of constipation. Factors such as a low-fiber diet, inadequate fluid intake, lack of physical activity, certain medications, and stress can contribute to this gastrointestinal trouble. Recognizing these triggers can help individuals make informed choices and develop a personalized plan to maintain regularity.

The Role of Nutrition

One of the most impactful ways to manage constipation is through dietary choices. A diet rich in fiber plays a pivotal role in promoting bowel health. Here are key nutritional strategies to incorporate:

Increase Fiber Intake:
Soluble Fiber: Found in oats, legumes, apples, and citrus fruits, soluble fiber absorbs water in the intestines, forming a gel-like substance that helps soften stools.
Insoluble Fiber: Present in whole grains, nuts, seeds, and vegetables, insoluble fiber adds bulk to the stool, facilitating its passage through the digestive tract.
Aim for a daily fiber intake of 25-30 grams. Gradually increasing fiber can prevent bloating and gas.

Stay Hydrated: Adequate hydration is critical for digestive health. Water helps dissolve soluble fiber, allowing it to work effectively. A general guideline is to drink at least eight 8-ounce glasses of water a day, but individual needs may vary based on activity level and climate.

Probiotic-Rich Foods: Incorporate foods that are high in probiotics, such as yogurt, kefir, sauerkraut,kimchi, and kombucha. These foods promote a healthy gut microbiome, which can enhance digestion and improve bowel regularity.

Mindful Eating: Paying attention to meal times can encourage regular bowel habits. Establishing a routine where meals are consumed at consistent times each day can help signal the body's digestive system to function optimally.

Physical Activity

Regular physical activity is essential for maintaining healthy bowel function. Exercise promotes motility in the digestive tract, preventing stagnation. Engaging in activities that elevate the heart rate and strengthen the core can be particularly beneficial. Here are some recommendations:

Daily Walks: Aim for at least 30 minutes of moderate-intensity aerobic exercise, whether throughbrisk walking, cycling, or swimming. This stimulates intestinal contractions.

Strength Training: Incorporate strength exercises two to three times a week. Muscle strength improvesoverall metabolism and can aid in digestion.

Yoga and Stretching: Certain yoga poses (such as

Child's Pose, Cat-Cow, and Seated Forward Bend) specifically stimulate the digestive organs and alleviate stress, a common contributor to constipation.

Stress Management

Stress and anxiety can significantly impact digestive health, leading to irregular bowel movements. Incorporating stress management techniques into your daily routine can improve gut function:

Mindfulness and Meditation: Practicing mindfulness meditation for as little as 10 to 15 minutes a daycan help reduce anxiety levels and improve overall emotional well-being.

Deep Breathing Exercises: Simple breathing techniques can promote relaxation and assist in managing stress, aiding in the prevention of stress-induced constipation.

Developing a Routine

Establishing a daily routine can be a powerful tool in managing constipation:

Morning Ritual: Start your day with a glass of warm water with lemon or herbal tea. This can stimulate digestion and signal to your body that it's time to move.

Scheduled Bathroom Breaks: Encourage regular bowel movements by setting aside time after meals, when the gastrocolic reflex (the natural urge to defecate following food intake) is strongest.

Listen to Your Body: Respond promptly to urges to go. Ignoring the signal can lead to a cycle of constipation.

While occasional constipation is normal for many individuals, chronic issues may require further medical evaluation. By taking proactive steps, individuals can empower themselves towards greater digestive health and overall well-being.

Chapter 7: Week 4 - Supporting Cleansing for Constipation Control with Chia Seeds

As we enter Week 4 of our transformative journey toward better health and well-being, it's time to delve into a natural and powerful solution for one of the most common digestive issues: constipation. In this chapter, we will explore how incorporating chia seeds into our diet can support cleansing processes, alleviate constipation, and promote overall digestive health.

Understanding Constipation

Constipation is a widespread condition characterized by

infrequent bowel movements, difficulty passing stools, or a sensation of incomplete evacuation. It can be caused by various factors, including inadequate fiber intake, dehydration, a sedentary lifestyle, and stress. The discomfort associated with constipation can lead to a feeling of heaviness and lethargy, negatively impacting our quality of life.

To effectively combat constipation, we must nourish our bodies by providing essential nutrients and maintaining digestive regularity. Natural remedies have gained popularity for their gentle yet effective approaches, one of which is the small but mighty chia seed.

The Nutritional Power of Chia Seeds

Chia seeds, derived from the *Salvia hispanica* plant, have been recognized for their health benefits for centuries, dating back to ancient civilizations like the Aztecs and Mayans. These tiny seeds are an abundant source of nutrients, rich in:

Dietary Fiber: Chia seeds have an exceptionally high fiber content, with approximately 10 grams of fiber per two-tablespoon serving. This amount helps create a gel-like substance in the digestive tract, improving stool consistency and promoting regular bowel movements.

Omega-3 Fatty Acids: These essential fatty acids support overall health, including reducing inflammation and promoting heart health. They also act as lubricants in the digestive tract, facilitating the passage of stools.

Protein: Chia seeds are a good source of plant-based protein, which is essential for muscle health and tissue repair, and can be beneficial during the detoxification process.

Vitamins and Minerals: Chia seeds contain important nutrients such as calcium, magnesium, and phosphorus, which contribute to optimal digestive functioning and play a role in maintaining overall health.

Chia Seeds as a Natural Lubricant

One of the primary mechanisms through which chia seeds help alleviate constipation is their ability to absorb water and form a gel-like substance. When chia seeds are mixed with liquid, they can absorb up to 12 times their weight, resulting in a highly viscous gel. This gel not only adds bulk to the stool but also provides lubrication, making it easier to pass.

Incorporating Chia Seeds into Your Diet

Now that we understand how chia seeds can support cleansing and aid in constipation control, let's explore various ways to incorporate them into our daily meals:

1. Chia Pudding

A delicious and versatile way to enjoy chia seeds is by making chia pudding. Combine 1/4 cup of chia seeds with 1 cup of milk (dairy or plant-based) and let it rest in the refrigerator overnight. In the morning, add fruits, nuts, or natural sweeteners to enhance the flavor and nutritional value.

2. Smoothies

Add a tablespoon of chia seeds to your favorite smoothie recipe. They blend easily into the mix and provide an extra boost of fiber and omega-3s without altering the flavor.

3. Baking

Incorporate chia seeds into baked goods such as breads, muffins, and pancakes. They can be added to recipes as a whole or ground into a powder for a subtler texture.

4. Salads and Soups

Sprinkle chia seeds on salads or stir them into soups for added crunch and nourishment. They can absorb the flavors of dressings and broths, enhancing the overall taste of your meals.

5. Hydration Boosters

For a refreshing drink, mix chia seeds with water, lemon juice, and a touch of honey. Let the mixture sit for about 10-15 minutes until the chia seeds expand, creating a satisfying and hydrating beverage.

Staying Hydrated

While chia seeds are an excellent source of dietary fiber, it's crucial to remember that adequate hydration is essential for their benefits to work effectively. Consuming chia seeds without enough water can lead to further discomfort and a potential risk of bowel obstruction. It's recommended to drink plenty of fluids throughout the day to keep your digestive system running smoothly.

Mindful Eating and Lifestyle Choices

In addition to incorporating chia seeds into our diet, we must adopt mindful eating habits and maintain an active lifestyle. Taking time to chew food thoroughly, practicing portion control, and listening to our bodies' hunger signals are practices that enhance digestion and promote regularity. Regular physical activity, even in the form of moderate walking, can stimulate bowel function and further alleviate constipation.

As we wrap up Week 4, we embrace chia seeds as a powerful ally in our journey toward improved digestive health and constipation control. By harnessing their nutritional benefits, we not only support cleansing processes but also cultivate a deeper understanding of our body's needs.

Maintaining Transformational Momentum for Constipation Control with Chia Seeds

Finding an effective and sustainable method for managing constipation can greatly improve one's quality of life. One such method that has gained traction in recent years is the incorporation of chia seeds into the diet. These tiny seeds, rich in fiber and omega-3 fatty acids, have transformative potential in promoting digestive health. This chapter will explore how to maintain a consistent momentum with chia seed consumption for effective constipation control.

The Nutritional Powerhouse of Chia Seeds

Chia seeds (Salvia hispanica) are not only high in dietary fiber but also serve as an excellent source of nutrients that promote digestive health:

Fiber Content: One ounce (28 grams) of chia seeds contains approximately 10 grams of fiber, making them an exceptional source of this critical nutrient. Fiber facilitates bowel movements by adding bulk to the stool and promoting regularity.

Omega-3 Fatty Acids: Chia seeds are rich in alpha-linolenic acid (ALA), a type of omega-3 fatty acid that helps reduce inflammation in the gut, potentially alleviating symptoms of constipation.

Hydration: Chia seeds can absorb up to 12 times their weight in water, expanding significantly when soaked. This property not only helps with hydration but also serves as a natural laxative, promoting the passage of stool.

Nutritional Versatility: Chia seeds can be easily incorporated into various meals. From smoothies to salads, their mild flavor and gelatinous texture when hydrated make them a versatile addition to any diet.

Creating a Chia Seed Routine

To harness the full benefits of chia seeds for constipation control, establishing a daily routine is crucial. Here are steps to facilitate the maintenance of transformational momentum:

1. Start Gradually

For those new to chia seeds, it's important to start with a smaller amount—about 1 teaspoon (5 grams) daily—and gradually increase to the recommended serving of 1–2 tablespoons (15-30 grams) over time. This helps the digestive system adjust to the increased fiber intake and ensures a smoother transition.

2. Hydrate

Ensure adequate water intake when consuming chia seeds. As they absorb water, the seeds expand. Consuming them without proper hydration may lead to digestive discomfort. Aim for at least 8-10 glasses ofwater each day to keep your digestive system moving smoothly.

3. Experiment with Preparation

Chia seeds can be consumed in various forms. Some popular methods include:

Chia Pudding: Mix chia seeds with almond milk, coconut milk, or yogurt. Let the mixture sit overnight in the refrigerator to thicken into a pudding. Add fruits, nuts, or honey for flavor and additionalnutrients.

Smoothies: Blend chia seeds into your favorite smoothies for a nutritious boost. They can be addedwhole or blended, depending on personal preference.

Baking: Incorporate chia seeds into baked goods like muffins, breads, and granola bars for addedfiber.

4. Monitor Response

As with any dietary change, it's essential to pay attention to how your body responds. Keep a journal to track your chia seed intake along with your digestive health, noting any changes in bowel regularity, comfort levels, or any adverse effects. This log can help in adjusting the daily intake to suit personal needs.

5. Combine with Other Fibers

Enhance the effectiveness of chia seeds by combining them with other sources of dietary fiber. Fruits and vegetables such as apples, pears, broccoli, and whole grains are excellent companions to chia seeds. This combination can create a synergistic effect, further promoting digestive health.

Educating Yourself and Others

Part of maintaining momentum is educating oneself about the health benefits of chia seeds. Understanding their nutritional profile and digestive advantages can encourage commitment to incorporating them into daily life. Furthermore, sharing knowledge with friends, family, and online communities can spread awareness and motivate others to explore this simple yet effective solution for constipation control.

Addressing Challenges

While chia seeds can be transformational, some

individuals may face challenges in integrating them into their diet. Common issues include:

Digestive Discomfort: If there are symptoms of bloating or gas, consider reducing the dosagetemporarily and increasing water intake.

Taste Preferences: Chia seeds have a subtle flavor. Recreational culinary exploration can help find enjoyable ways to consume them, such as infusing them in flavored water or incorporating them into savorydishes.

Maintaining Consistency: Life can become busy, so consider prepping chia puddings or smoothies inadvance to simplify meal preparation and ensure consistent intake.

Maintaining transformational momentum for constipation control through the incorporation of chia seeds can lead to substantial improvements in digestive health.

Transitioning to Long-Term Health of the body with chia seeds

Small yet mighty, these tiny seeds boast a wealth of nutrients that can significantly impact our overall well-being. This chapter explores how incorporating chia seeds into our daily lives can facilitate a seamless transition to long-term health, emphasizing gradual changes, sustainable practices, and diverse applications.

The Nutritional Powerhouse of Chia Seeds

Chia seeds, derived from the Salvia hispanica plant, are rich in omega-3 fatty acids, antioxidants, fiber, protein, and a variety of essential micronutrients. Just two tablespoons (approximately 28 grams) of chia seeds can provide:

Omega-3 Fatty Acids: Promotes heart health and reduces inflammation.
Fiber: Aids digestion and promotes satiety, helping in weight management.
Protein: Supports muscle repair and overall bodily functions.
Calcium, Magnesium, and Iron: Essential for bone health, energy production, and red blood cell formation.

These components make chia seeds a valuable addition to a balanced diet, serving as a foundation upon which to build long-term health.

The Science Behind Chia Seeds and Health

Research suggests that regular consumption of chia seeds may contribute to numerous health benefits, including:

Heart Health: Omega-3 fatty acids are known to lower blood pressure, reduce cholesterol levels, and improve heart rhythm. By incorporating chia seeds into your diet, you can take proactive steps toward cardiovascular wellness.

Digestive Health: The fiber content in chia seeds helps maintain proper digestive function, preventing constipation and promoting gut health. It also supports the growth of beneficial gut bacteria.

Weight Management: Chia seeds expand when mixed with liquid, which can help promote feelings of fullness, reducing overall caloric intake. This property can be particularly beneficial for those looking to maintain a healthy weight.

Blood Sugar Regulation: Studies indicate that chia seeds may improve insulin sensitivity and lower blood sugar levels, which is vital for those managing diabetes or seeking to prevent it.

Transitioning into the Chia Seed Lifestyle

Transitioning to a diet rich in chia seeds does not have to be overwhelming. Here are some practical tips for incorporating chia seeds into your long-term health regimen:

1. Start Small

Begin with one tablespoon of chia seeds daily. You can mix them into yogurt, smoothies, or oatmeal. Gradually increasing your intake allows your body to adjust to the added fiber without causing discomfort.

2. Explore Recipes

There are countless ways to incorporate chia seeds into your meals. Consider trying:

Chia Pudding: Combine chia seeds with your favorite milk or milk alternative, sweetener, and flavorings (vanilla, cocoa, spices) and refrigerate overnight for a nutritious breakfast or snack.

Chia Jam: Blend fruits with chia seeds to create a healthy, homemade jam. The chia seeds will thicken the mixture, creating a delicious spread.

Baked Goods: Add chia seeds to muffins, breads, or pancakes for an extra nutritional boost.

3. Stay Hydrated
Chia seeds absorb up to ten times their weight in water. It's crucial to drink plenty of fluids throughout the day, especially when consuming chia seeds, to aid digestion and prevent any potential discomfort.

4. Combine with Other Superfoods
Maximize their benefits by pairing chia seeds with other nutrient-dense foods, such as berries, nuts, and leafy greens. This combination ensures you're getting a wide array of vitamins and minerals essential for long- term health.

5. Monitor Your Body's Response

As you introduce chia seeds into your diet, pay attention to how your body reacts. Everyone is different, and it may take time to see and feel the benefits. Keep a journal to track your energy levels, digestive health, and overall well-being.

The Mindset of Healthy Living

Embracing a lifestyle that prioritizes long-term health requires a shift in mindset. Rather than focusing solely on immediate results, cultivate an appreciation for the gradual, sustainable changes that accompany a balanced diet rich in superfoods like chia seeds. Set realistic goals, celebrate small victories, and recognize that health is a journey, not a destination.

Transitioning to long-term health using chia seeds is a manageable and rewarding process. By understanding the nutritional benefits of chia seeds, embracing practical incorporation techniques, and fostering a mindset geared toward sustainable living, one can lay a strong foundation for overall health and wellness.

Chapter 8: Lifestyle Tips for Regularity ofConstipation Control

Although it may seem like a minor annoyance, the discomfort and potential health consequences it brings can be significant. Fortunately, many lifestyle changes can help effectively manage and alleviate constipation. In this chapter, we will explore practical tips and strategies that can lead to better bowel regularity and overall digestive health.

Understanding Constipation

Before diving into lifestyle tips, it's essential to understand what constipation is. Constipation is typically characterized by infrequent bowel movements, difficulty passing stools, or a sensation of incomplete evacuation. Contributing factors include poor dietary habits, lack of physical activity, inadequate hydration, and stress. By addressing these factors, one can develop a more consistent and effective routine for intestinal health.

1. Dietary Adjustments

Increase Fiber Intake

One of the most effective ways to combat constipation is to increase dietary fiber. Fiber adds bulk to the stool and promotes peristalsis, the wave-like movements that move food through the digestive tract. Foods high in fiber include:

Fruits and Vegetables: Apples, pears, berries, carrots, and leafy greens.
Whole Grains: Oats, brown rice, quinoa, and whole grain bread.

Legumes: Beans, lentils, and chickpeas.

Aim for a daily fiber intake of 25 to 30 grams. Incorporating a variety of types of fiber (soluble, found in oats and fruits, and insoluble, found in whole grains and vegetables) can optimize digestive health.

Stay Hydrated

Proper hydration is crucial for maintaining bowel regularity. Water helps dissolve soluble fiber and facilitates the movement of waste through the intestines. Try to drink at least eight 8-ounce glasses (about 2 liters) of water a day. If you are physically active or live in a warm climate, you may need even more. Consider incorporating herbal teas and hydrating fruits like watermelon or cucumbers into your diet.

2. Regular Physical Activity

Exercise Routine

Sedentary behavior can contribute to constipation. Regular physical activity stimulates digestion and promotes bowel regularity. Aim for at least 150 minutes of moderate aerobic activity each week, such as brisk walking, cycling, or swimming. You should also include muscle-strengthening exercises at least twice a week.

Specific Exercises
Certain exercises can be particularly effective in promoting bowel movement:

Walking: A simple walk after meals can stimulate digestion.
Yoga: Poses like the forward bend, seated twist, and

child's pose can relieve tension and improve bowel function.

Pelvic Floor Exercises: Strengthening the pelvic floor muscles through exercises like Kegels can enhance control during bowel movements.
3. Establish a Routine ### Optimize Bowel Habits
Developing a consistent routine can significantly improve bowel regularity. Here are a few actionable tips to create a routine:

Set Scheduled Times: Try to go to the bathroom at the same times each day, preferably after a meal when the digestive system is most active.
Don't Ignore Urges: When you feel the urge to have a bowel movement, respond promptly. Ignoring these signals can lead to constipation over time.

Create a Relaxing Environment
A calm and comfortable bathroom environment can encourage relaxation and facilitate bowel movements. Consider:

Having Privacy: Ensure you have time alone to avoid feeling rushed.
Incorporating Comfort: Use a footstool to elevate the feet slightly while sitting, as this can help align the rectum and facilitate easier passage of stool.
Deep Breathing: Take a few deep breaths to relax your body and reduce stress, which can impede bowel function.

4. Manage Stress

Mindfulness and Relaxation Techniques
Stress can be a significant contributor to constipation. Practicing mindfulness and relaxation techniques can mitigate its effects. Consider:

Meditation: Spend a few minutes each day focusing on your breath and clearing your mind.
Yoga and Stretching: Incorporating gentle yoga stretches can alleviate tension in the body and promote circulation.
Journaling: Writing down thoughts and feelings can help manage stress and contribute to emotional well-being.

5. Consult Healthcare Professionals

If lifestyle changes do not improve constipation symptoms or if you experience severe discomfort, it may be time to consult with a healthcare professional. They can provide guidance, recommend appropriate treatments, or rule out underlying conditions.

Managing constipation doesn't have to be complicated. By making mindful dietary choices, staying active, establishing regular routines, managing stress, and seeking professional advice when needed, you can take control of your digestive health. Remember, consistency is key.

Specific Exercise and Physical Activity to Reduce Constipation

While various factors contribute to constipation, including diet, hydration, and medications, physical activity is a key component that can promote gastrointestinal health and stimulate bowel function. This chapter will explore specific exercises and physical activities that can help alleviate constipation, highlighting their physiological benefits as well as practical recommendations for incorporation into daily routines.

Understanding the Physiology of Constipation

The human digestive system relies on a coordinated effort between the muscles of the intestines and the nervous system. When food enters the intestines, a process known as peristalsis occurs—waves of muscle contractions push food through the digestive tract. Sedentary lifestyles can lead to sluggish movements within the intestines, contributing to a higher risk of constipation. Exercise enhances blood circulation, stimulates muscle contractions, and helps maintain a healthy weight, all of which can have a positive impact on bowel regularity.

The Role of Exercise in Digestive Health

Increased Bowel Motility: Physical activity activates the enteric nervous system, which controls digestive processes. Exercise can stimulate contractions in the intestines, allowing for more efficient transportation of waste.

Strengthening Core Muscles: Exercises that strengthen the abdominal and core muscles can help improve posture and support the proper functioning of the digestive system.

Relieving Stress and Anxiety: Mental health plays a significant role in gastrointestinal health.Regular physical activity has been shown to reduce stress and anxiety, factors that can exacerbate constipation.

Improving Overall Health: Maintaining a healthy weight through exercise can also worsen constipation; obesity is associated with an increased risk of gastrointestinal disorders, including constipation.

Specific Exercises to Alleviate Constipation

Here are several specific exercise modalities and types of physical activity that can be effective in reducing constipation:

1. Aerobic Exercises

Aerobic activities, such as walking, running, cycling, and swimming, are excellent for stimulating bowelmovement. Aim for at least 150 minutes of moderate aerobic activity per week.

Walking: A brisk walk for 30 minutes daily can enhance digestive system performance. It contracts the abdominal muscles, promoting bowel movements.

Cycling: Whether on a stationary bike or cycling outdoors, pedaling is a low-impact way to stimulate digestion.

2. Strength Training

Resistance exercises can also play a role in digestive health. Strengthening the abdominal muscles helps create the muscular foundation necessary for efficient peristalsis.

Bodyweight Exercises: Squats, lunges, and planks engage core muscles directly and support metabolic activity.

Weightlifting: Incorporating tools like dumbbells or resistance bands can increase the intensity and effectiveness of your workouts.

3. Yoga

Yoga is not only beneficial for flexibility and balance but also incredibly helpful for digestion.

Poses for Digestion: Try poses such as the "Cat-Cow," "Seated Forward Bend," or "Twists" which can massage the intestines and stimulate circulation.

Breathwork: Deep breathing techniques practiced in yoga can help reduce stress and promote relaxation, both of which aid in digestion.

4. Stretching and Mobility Exercises

Gentle stretching and mobility work can support digestive health by encouraging blood flow and relieving tension in the abdomen.

Dynamic Stretching: Incorporate movements such as torso twists or side stretches which can engage the abdominal area.

Foam Rolling: This technique can alleviate tightness in the fascia surrounding the intestines, encouraging better blood flow and mobility.

Practical Recommendations for Incorporating Exercise

Set Realistic Goals: Start with manageable durations and intensity levels, gradually increasing as your fitness improves.

Establish a Routine: Consistency is key to reaping the benefits of physical activity. Aim to incorporate exercise into your daily routine, such as walking after meals, which can aid digestion.

Stay Hydrated: Pairing exercise with adequate hydration is essential for digestive health. Make sure to drink plenty of water before, during, and after physical activity.

Listen to Your Body: Pay attention to how your body responds to different exercises. Some individuals may find certain movements more beneficial than others.

Seek Professional Guidance: If you're unsure about which exercises are appropriate for you, consulting a personal trainer or physical therapist can provide personalized recommendations tailored to your needs.

Combining specific exercises and physical activity into your daily routine can significantly reduce the incidence and severity of constipation. Through a better understanding of the physiological mechanisms and the incorporation of various movement modalities—from aerobic exercise to yoga—individuals can actively participate in their digestive health.

Stress Management and Sleep

Whether from work, relationships, or personal responsibilities, stress levels can easily escalate, leading to a myriad of physical and mental health issues. One of the most significant impacts of chronic stress is its effect on sleep quality and duration. In this chapter, we will explore the complex relationship between stress and sleep, highlighting effective strategies for stress management that can enhance sleep quality.

The Connection Between Stress and Sleep

Sleep is a natural restorative process essential for maintaining physical health and emotional well-being. However, stress can disrupt this process in several ways. When faced with stress, our bodies produce higher levels of cortisol, the primary stress hormone. Elevated cortisol levels can lead to insomnia, interrupted sleep patterns, and a reduction in the amount of restorative deep sleep we experience.

Moreover, stress often triggers racing thoughts, anxiety, and restlessness, making it challenging to relax and fall asleep. The cycle of stress affecting sleep, and inadequate sleep leading to increased stress, creates a vicious cycle that can be hard to break. Recognizing this connection is the first step in managing stress to improve sleep quality.

Identifying Stress Triggers

The first step in managing stress is to identify what triggers it. Common sources of stress include:

Work-related pressures: Deadlines, workload, and job security can induce significant stress.
Personal relationships: Conflicts with family, friends, or partners can weigh heavily on the mind.
Financial concerns: Worries about bills, debt, or budgeting can lead to anxiety.
Life changes: Major life events, such as moving, getting married, or having a child, can be both joyous and stressful.
Health issues: Chronic health problems, either personal or within the family, can create ongoing stress.

Keeping a stress journal can help identify patterns and triggers, empowering individuals to address the sources of their stress directly.

Effective Stress Management Techniques

Once you understand your stress triggers, it's essential to develop effective management techniques. Here are several strategies that can help:

1. Mindfulness and Meditation

Mindfulness involves being fully present in the moment without judgment. Practicing mindfulness or meditation regularly can significantly reduce stress levels by promoting relaxation and enhancing overall well-being. Even a few minutes of mindfulness each day can help calm the mind and prepare it for restful sleep.

2. Physical Activity

Exercise is a powerful stress reliever. Engaging in regular physical activity releases endorphins, which improve mood and promote feelings of well-being. Whether it's walking, yoga, or a more vigorous workout, finding an enjoyable form of exercise can reduce stress and prepare your body for a good night's sleep.

3. Healthy Sleep Hygiene

Establishing good sleep hygiene can greatly improve sleep quality. Consider the following practices:

Create a sleep schedule: Go to bed and wake up at the same time each day, even on weekends.
Limit screen time: Reduce exposure to screens at least an hour before bedtime to minimize blue light interference with melatonin production.
Create a calming bedtime routine: Engage in relaxing activities like reading or taking a warm bath before bed.
Make your sleeping environment comfortable: Ensure your bedroom is conducive to sleep with a comfortable

mattress, suitable temperature, and minimal noise and light.

4. Healthy Diet

Nutrition plays a key role in both stress levels and sleep quality. Avoid excessive caffeine and sugar, especially later in the day. Instead, opt for a balanced diet rich in fruits, vegetables, lean proteins, and wholegrains. Foods high in magnesium, such as leafy greens and nuts, can also help promote relaxation.

5. Seek Support

Talk to friends, family, or professionals about your stress. Sharing your feelings can provide relief and offer new perspectives on managing stressors. Support groups or therapy can also be excellent resources for coping strategies.

The Importance of Routine

Establishing a regular routine can provide structure in times of stress. Designate time each day for relaxation, exercise, and supportive relationships. Routines create predictability, which can help alleviate feelings of chaos during stressful periods.

Stress and sleep are intricately linked, and managing one can significantly improve the other. By actively identifying stress triggers, employing effective stress management techniques, and prioritizing healthy sleep hygiene, individuals can break the cycle of stress and poor sleep.

Chapter 9: Long-Term Health and Wellness

This chapter delves into the pillars of long-term wellness, emphasizing the importance of a holistic approach that encompasses physical, mental, and emotional health.

Understanding Long-Term Health

Long-term health refers to maintaining a balanced state of physical and mental well-being over an extended period. It is not simply the absence of disease but rather an ongoing process of growth and development that allows individuals to thrive. This multifaceted nature of health involves several interconnected dimensions:

1. Physical Health

Physical health serves as the cornerstone of overall well-being. It encompasses regular exercise, a balanced diet, adequate rest, and routine health check-ups. Long-term physical health is achieved through:

Regular Exercise: Engaging in physical activity not only promotes cardiovascular health but also improves muscular strength, flexibility, and endurance. Finding an enjoyable exercise routine—whether it's dancing, hiking, swimming, or practicing yoga—can make maintaining an active lifestyle enjoyable.

Nutrition: Fueling the body with the right nutrients is essential for maintaining energy levels and preventing chronic diseases. A diet rich in fruits, vegetables, whole grains, lean proteins, and healthy fats can significantly impact how we feel and function.

Sleep Hygiene: The importance of quality sleep for health is often underestimated. Establishing a consistent sleep schedule and creating a calm environment can greatly enhance overall health and mental clarity.

2. Mental and Emotional Well-Being

Mental and emotional well-being is just as important as physical health, encompassing the ability to manage stress, maintain relationships, and adapt to change. Long-term strategies include:

Mindfulness and Stress Management: Practices such as meditation, deep breathing exercises, or engaging in hobbies can help reduce stress and promote a state of calm. Recognizing stress triggers and finding effective coping mechanisms is crucial for mental resilience.

Social Connections: Building and maintaining meaningful relationships can provide emotional support and enhance feelings of belonging. Regularly connecting with family and friends and participating in social activities can strengthen emotional and mental health.

Therapeutic Support: Seeking professional help when needed is essential. Therapy can provide tools to navigate life's challenges, build emotional intelligence, and foster personal growth.

3. Preventive Healthcare

Preventive healthcare plays a critical role in long-term health. Regular screenings, vaccinations, and health assessments help detect potential health issues before they become serious. Engaging with healthcare professionals and being proactive about health choices empowers individuals to take control of their well- being.

Developing Healthy Habits

Building long-lasting health habits requires conscious effort and commitment. Here are some strategies to foster healthy practices:

1. Goal Setting

Establishing specific, measurable, attainable, relevant, and time-bound (SMART) goals can serve as a powerful motivator. Whether aiming to lose weight, improve stamina, or cultivate a new skill, setting clear objectives can help in tracking progress and maintaining focus.

2. Consistency over Perfection

Embracing a mindset of consistency rather than perfection encourages sustainable change. It is better to incorporate manageable health practices into daily life rather than striving for an unattainable ideal.

Fostering a growth mindset allows for setbacks to be seen as opportunities for learning rather than failures.

3. Education and Awareness
Staying informed about health and wellness trends, nutrition labels, and the importance of physical activity empowers individuals to make informed choices. Knowledge is a vital component in cultivating a culture of health.

In this journey, taking small, conscious steps can lead to monumental changes, transforming short-term efforts into lifelong habits of health. As we conclude this chapter, remember that the path to long-term wellness is a continuous journey, one that can bring profound rewards to those brave enough to embark upon it.

Creating a Sustainable Routine

Today, the focus is not just on sustainable practices but on creating a sustainable routine that can lead to a more balanced, fulfilling lifestyle. This chapter aims to explore the foundational principles of a sustainable routine, provide practical steps to develop one, and highlight the benefits of integrating these practices into your everyday life.

Understanding Sustainable Routines

A sustainable routine is one that supports long-term well-being without depleting your physical, mental, or emotional resources. Just as we must consider the environmental impact of our actions, we should also recognize the significance of our habits on our personal health and happiness. The goal is to create a routine that allows for growth, reduces stress, and aligns with your core values.

The Principles of a Sustainable Routine

Balance: A sustainable routine requires a balance

between work, rest, and play. It's essential to set aside time for your responsibilities, self-care, and leisure activities that recharge you.

Flexibility: Life is unpredictable, and a rigid routine can lead to stress when unexpected events arise. A sustainable practice allows flexibility, enabling you to adapt without losing sight of your goals.

Mindfulness: Being aware of your choices and their impacts is crucial. Mindfulness helps you stay present, making it easier to prioritize activities that nourish your body, mind, and spirit.

Simplicity: Keep your routine simple. Overloading your schedule can lead to burnout. Focus on essential activities that bring you joy and fulfillment.

Intentionality: Every action in a sustainable routine should be intentional. Identify your goals and ensure each activity aligns with your long-term objectives and values.

Steps to Create Your Sustainable Routine

Creating a sustainable routine requires thoughtful planning and experimentation. Here are steps to help you craft a routine that works for you:

Step 1: Self-Assessment

Begin by assessing your current routine. Take note of how you spend your time, what makes you feel energized, and what drains you. Journaling for a week can help reveal patterns in your daily activities.

Step 2: Identify Priorities

Once you have a clear picture of your habits, identify your priorities. What matters most to you? Consider aspects such as health, relationships, career aspirations, personal growth, and leisure. Grab a notepad and list these values, then rank them in order of importance.

Step 3: Set Realistic Goals

Based on your priorities, set realistic and achievable goals. Instead of vague aspirations like "get healthy," specify measurable targets, like "exercise for 30 minutes three times a week." This clarity will guide your daily actions.

Step 4: Plan Your Routine

With your goals in mind, start mapping out your routine. Consider using time-blocking techniques, which involve dividing your day into chunks dedicated to specific tasks or activities. Remember to incorporate breaks, exercise, family time, and leisure activities that bring you joy.

Step 5: Integrate Self-Care

In a sustainable routine, self-care must take center stage. Schedule regular time for activities that recharge your energy—whether it's reading a book, practicing yoga, or spending time with loved ones. Prioritize sleepas well, as adequate rest is essential for maintaining overall health.

Step 6: Evaluate and Adjust

No routine is set in stone. Regularly evaluate what's working and what isn't. Are you feeling overwhelmed? Do you feel fulfilled and balanced? Adjust your schedule as needed to better suit your needs and circumstances.

The Benefits of a Sustainable Routine

Improved Well-Being: A well-balanced routine can enhance your physical and mental health, reducing stress and promoting happiness.

Increased Productivity: By focusing your energy on well-defined priorities, you can improve yourproductivity in both personal and professional realms.

Enhanced Relationships: Allocating time for family and friends fosters deeper connections and support systems critical for emotional well-being.

Personal Growth: A sustainable routine encourages continuous learning and self-discovery, allowing you to pursue your passions and interests.

Environmental Awareness: As you cultivate mindfulness, you're likely to become more aware of how your choices affect the environment, leading to a more sustainable lifestyle.

Creating a sustainable routine is an evolving process that requires patience and commitment. By embracing balance, flexibility, and intentionality, you can forge a path toward a lifestyle that nurtures your well-being and aligns with your values.

Celebrating Your Success in Reducing Constipation with Chia Seeds

For many, digestive issues, particularly constipation, can be a source of discomfort and frustration. However, as we delve into the life-changing benefits of chia seeds, it's essential to pause and recognize the strides you've made in promoting your digestive health. This chapter celebrates your success in reducing constipation with chia seeds—a tiny yet powerful addition to your diet.

Understanding Constipation and Natural Remedies

Before we delve into your achievements, it's crucial to understand the landscape of constipation. Defined as infrequent or difficult bowel movements, constipation affects millions worldwide. The causes range from dietary choices to lifestyle habits and even stress levels. Conventional remedies—laxatives, fiber supplements, or over-the-counter medications—often come with side effects, prompting many to seek natural solutions.

Chia seeds, derived from the Salvia hispanica plant, have emerged as a nutritional powerhouse, boasting high fiber content, omega-3 fatty acids, protein, and essential vitamins and minerals. Their unique ability to absorb water, swelling up to ten times their original size, enhances their effectiveness in alleviating constipation and promoting regular bowel movements.

The Journey Towards Digestive Health

Your journey towards improved digestive health likely wasn't instantaneous. Initially, you may have felt hesitant to make changes in your diet or reluctant to try chia seeds, questioning their efficacy. Perhaps you struggled with feelings of discomfort from constipation, impacting your mood and daily activities. However, with determination and a commitment to your health, you began incorporating chia seeds into your meals and snacks, slowly witnessing a change.

Small Steps Lead to Big Changes

The beauty of using chia seeds lies in their versatility. Whether you blended them into your morning smoothie, sprinkled them over a fresh salad, or mixed them into your favorite yogurt, every tiny seed you consumed brought you a step closer to digestive relief. Perhaps you celebrated small victories as the days went by—those moments when the uncomfortable tightness in your abdomen subsided, or the ease of your bowel movements increased dramatically.

As you incorporated chia seeds, you may have assembled a repertoire of delectable recipes that aligned with your lifestyle. From chia puddings bursting with flavor to hearty chia energy bars, these nutritious options ensured that you did not feel deprived while taking control of your health.

Acknowledging the Power of Hydration

Chia seeds are best known for their gel-like consistency when hydrated, making their pairing with water or other fluids essential for optimal results. By prioritizing hydration alongside your chia seed intake, you discovered a pivotal connection between water consumption and digestive health. This mindful habit served to enhance the seeds' natural effectiveness and furthered your ability to maintain a balanced digestive system.

The Tangible Results

As your perseverance paid off, you began to notice tangible results. Perhaps you found yourself sharing these wins with friends and family, delighting in your newfound energy and overall sense of well-being. Better digestion opens up a realm of opportunity—be it going out without fear of discomfort or embracing spontaneous meals without anxiety.

With chia seeds supporting your diet, you learned the power of listening to your body. You became attuned to what foods nourished you, recognizing the connection between your dietary choices and how they translated into wellness.

Creating a Community of Support

In navigating your journey, you may have engaged with others in your sphere—friends, family, or online communities—sharing your experiences and perhaps offering advice to those grappling with similar issues. By celebrating your successes, you have contributed to a culture of awareness surrounding gut health and the natural remedies available, encouraging others to consider dietary changes that promote well-being.

This ripple effect not only fosters support but also reinforces your victories. Each discussion and shared recipe becomes a beacon of hope and encouragement for others, and together, you celebrate not merely individual triumphs, but collective progress in understanding and managing digestive health.

Looking Ahead

As we conclude this chapter, take a moment to reflect on your journey. You have empowered yourself by making informed choices and embracing the healing potential of nature's bounty. Your success in reducing constipation with chia seeds is not just a personal victory, but a celebration of a healthier lifestyle overall.

Moving forward, consider how you can continue to build on this foundation of success. Perhaps experiment with complementary foods rich in fiber, such as fruits, vegetables, and whole grains, or explore other natural remedies that align with your health goals. Each step is an invitation to cultivate a compassionate relationship with your body—a chance to celebrate every small victory in your journey toward optimal health.

In the grand tapestry of life, let this be a moment to commemorate your achievements, shine a spotlight on your resilience, and emerge with the confidence that you possess the tools needed to nurture your well-being and that of those around you. With every scoop of chia seeds, you are not just nourishing your body; you are honoring your journey toward health and happiness. Cheers to you and the vibrant life that awaits!

Chapter 10: Chia Seeds and Hydration

In this chapter, we will explore the origins of chia seeds, their nutritional benefits, and how they can play a crucial role in maintaining optimal hydration levels.

The Origins of Chia Seeds

Chia seeds (Salvia hispanica) have their roots in ancient Mesoamerica, where they were a staple food for the Aztecs and Mayans. These small black or white seeds were revered not only for their nutritional contributions but also for their ability to provide sustained energy. The name "chia" comes from the Mayan word meaning "strength," highlighting its historical importance as a source of fuel for warriors and travelers alike.

Nutritional Benefits of Chia Seeds

Chia seeds are a powerhouse of nutritional energy. They are packed with essential nutrients, making them a valuable addition to any diet. Just one ounce (approximately two tablespoons) contains about:

Fiber: Chia seeds are an excellent source of dietary fiber, with nearly 10 grams per ounce. This fiber content aids digestion, promotes a feeling of fullness, and helps regulate blood sugar levels.

Omega-3 Fatty Acids: They are among the best plant sources of omega-3 fatty acids, particularly alpha-linolenic acid (ALA). Omega-3s are crucial for heart health, brain function, and reducing inflammation in the body.

Protein: Chia seeds contain about 20% protein, making them an excellent option for vegetarians and vegans looking to increase their protein intake. They provide all nine essential amino acids, which are vital for muscle repair and growth.

Vitamins and Minerals: Chia seeds are rich in several important nutrients, including calcium, magnesium, phosphorus, and antioxidants, all of which contribute to overall health and well-being.

Chia Seeds and Hydration

One of the most fascinating properties of chia seeds is their ability to absorb liquids. When soaked in water or any other liquid, chia seeds can expand up to 12 times their original size, forming a gel-like consistency. This remarkable absorption capacity is key to understanding how chia seeds can enhance hydration.

How Do Chia Seeds Promote Hydration?

Water Absorption: Chia seeds can retain significant amounts of water, helping to create a reservoir of hydration in the body. When consumed, they can slow down digestion and provide a lasting source of moisture.

Electrolyte Balance: Chia seeds contain important electrolytes such as potassium and sodium, which are essential for maintaining fluid balance in the body. This balance is crucial, especially during exercise or in hot climates, where dehydration can occur rapidly.

Sustained Energy Release: The combination of fiber, protein, and healthy fats in chia seeds provides a steady energy release, helping to prolong hydration levels. People who consume chia seeds may find that they feel fuller longer, reducing the tendency to snack on dehydrating foods.

How to Incorporate Chia Seeds for Hydration

Incorporating chia seeds into your diet doesn't have to be complicated. Here are several simple and delicious ways to enjoy them while boosting your hydration:

Chia Seed Pudding: Combine chia seeds with milk (dairy or plant-based) and a natural sweetener, letting the mixture sit overnight. In the morning, you'll have a nutritious pudding that is both hydrating andsatisfying.

Smoothies: Toss a tablespoon of chia seeds into your favorite smoothie. They'll blend well whileadding a thick texture and nutritional benefits.

Water Infusion: Soak chia seeds in water for about 10-15 minutes until they form a gel. Add this gel toflavored water or juice for a nutrient boost.

Baked Goods: Incorporate chia seeds into your baking recipes, such as muffins or bread, to enhance both hydration and nutritional content.

As we continue to uncover the many benefits of incorporating chia seeds into our diets, it becomes clear that they serve a dual purpose—providing essential nutrients while enhancing hydration. Their versatility and impressive health profile make them an ideal food for anyone looking to maintain optimal hydration levels ina world that often prioritizes convenience over nutrition.

Importance of Staying Hydrated for Constipation Control

Characterized by infrequent bowel movements, hard

stools, and discomfort, constipation can significantly impact an individual's quality of life. While many factors contribute to this condition, one of the most critical aspects of managing constipation is hydration. This chapter explores the significance of staying hydrated and how it plays a vital role in promoting digestive health and relieving constipation.

Understanding Constipation

Before delving into the relationship between hydration and constipation, it's essential to understand what constipation is. Generally defined as having fewer than three bowel movements per week, constipation can arise from various causes, including a low-fiber diet, sedentary lifestyle, certain medications, and dehydration. When the body lacks sufficient fluid, the colon pulls water from the waste material, leading to harder stools that are difficult to pass.

The Role of Water in Digestion

Water is crucial for numerous physiological processes, including digestion. It helps break down food so that the nutrients can be absorbed effectively. Water aids in dissolving vitamins, minerals, and other nutrients, allowing them to be transported throughout the body. Furthermore, adequate hydration ensures that the mucosal lining of the intestines remains moist, facilitating smoother bowel movements.

Hydration and Stool Consistency

One of the primary benefits of staying hydrated is its effect on stool consistency. When the body is well- hydrated, the stool retains more water, making it softer and easier to pass. On the contrary, dehydration leads to firm and dry stools, increasing the risk of constipation. The addition of water to the dietary fiber consumed helps to create a gel-like substance that promotes regular bowel movements. Therefore, a diet rich in both fiber and fluids is a cornerstone of effective constipation management.

Recommended Hydration Levels

The amount of water a person needs can vary based on various factors, including age, sex, activity level, and overall health. As a general guideline, health experts recommend drinking at least eight 8-ounce glasses of water a day—commonly referred to as the "8x8 rule." However, individuals with high physical activity levels or those living in hot climates may require more water. Additionally, other beverages, as well as foods with high water content, such as fruits and vegetables, can contribute to overall hydration.

Signs of Dehydration

Recognizing the signs of dehydration is crucial for preventing constipation. Early symptoms may include dry mouth, fatigue, headache, and dizziness. More severe dehydration can lead to reduced urine output, dark-colored urine, and confusion. By paying attention to these signs and increasing fluid intake, individuals can take proactive steps to prevent constipation and maintain overall gastrointestinal health.

Strategies for Staying Hydrated

Maintaining proper hydration can be challenging for some, especially in a fast-paced lifestyle. However, there are several simple strategies to ensure adequate fluid intake:

Carry a Water Bottle: Keeping a reusable water bottle on hand serves as a constant reminder to drink throughout the day. Aim to refill it regularly.

Set Reminders: Use smartphone apps or alarms to remind you to drink water hourly or at specific intervals.

Incorporate Hydrating Foods: Include fruits and vegetables like cucumbers, oranges, and strawberries in your diet. These foods not only provide hydration but also contribute vital nutrients.

Flavor Your Water: For those who find plain water unappealing, adding slices of lemon, cucumber, or mint can enhance the taste and encourage increased consumption.

Drink Before Meals: Make it a habit to drink a glass of water before each meal. This not only promotes hydration but can also help with portion control.

By understanding the relationship between hydration and bowel function, individuals can take proactive steps to improve their overall wellness. Implementing daily hydration strategies, recognizing the signs of dehydration, and enjoying the benefits of a well-hydrated body can lead to more regular bowel movements and enhance one's quality of life. As such, making hydration a priority is a small yet powerful step toward achieving better digestive health and constipation control.

How Chia Seeds Help with Body Hydration

As individuals increasingly seek natural ways to support hydration, superfoods like chia seeds have emerged as a powerful ally. This chapter will explore how chia seeds contribute to body hydration, their unique properties, and practical ways to incorporate them into your diet.

The Hydration Challenge

The human body is composed of approximately 60% water, which is vital for maintaining bodily functions and homeostasis. Hydration affects energy levels, skin health, digestion, and even mood. Despite its importance, many people struggle to consume adequate fluids daily. Factors such as busy lifestyles, physical activity, climate, and dietary habits can all affect hydration levels.

While drinking water is the most straightforward solution, incorporating foods rich in water content and electrolytes into our diets can also promote hydration. This is where chia seeds come into play.

Chia Seeds: A Nutritional Powerhouse

Chia seeds (Salvia hispanica) are tiny black or white seeds derived from the flowering plant native to Mexico and Guatemala. Packed with nutrients, chia seeds are an excellent source of fiber, protein, healthy fats, vitamins, and minerals. One of their most remarkable traits is their ability to absorb water—a quality that greatly enhances their potential as a hydrating food.

How Chia Seeds Promote Hydration

Water Absorption: Chia seeds have an extraordinary ability to absorb water, expanding up to 10-12 times their original size when soaked. This gel-like substance is formed when the soluble fiber in the seeds ismixed with water. When consumed, this gel can help retain moisture in the body longer, supporting hydration levels over time.

Slow Digestion: The high fiber content in chia seeds slows down the digestion process, resulting in agradual release of nutrients and water into the bloodstream. This slow absorption helps maintain hydration and keeps the feeling of fullness for longer durations, making them an excellent addition to meals or snacks.

Electrolyte Balance: In addition to their water-holding capacity, chia seeds contain essential mineralslike potassium, magnesium, and calcium, which are crucial for maintaining electrolyte balance. Proper electrolyte levels are pivotal for hydration, as they help regulate the distribution of fluids in the body.

Sustained Energy: Consuming chia seeds can provide a steady source of energy due to their balance of carbohydrates, protein, and fats. This energy source is particularly beneficial for athletes and active individuals who require prolonged hydration and stamina during physical activities.

Practical Ways to Incorporate Chia Seeds into Your Diet

Chia Pudding: One of the most popular ways to enjoy chia seeds is by making chia pudding. Combine chia seeds with your choice of milk (dairy or plant-based), sweetener, and flavorings such as vanilla or cocoa powder. Let it sit for a few hours or overnight until it thickens into a delicious pudding.

Smoothies: Add a tablespoon of chia seeds to your smoothies for an added boost of hydration and nutrition. The seeds will not only enhance the texture but also help keep you full and hydrated throughout the day.

Baked Goods: Incorporate chia seeds into muffins, bread, or energy bars. When baked, they add a nutritional punch without altering the flavor significantly.

Soups and Sauces: Thicken soups or sauces with soaked chia seeds instead of flour. This can enhance both the texture and nutrient profile of your meals.

Infused Water: For a refreshing drink, add chia seeds to infused water. Combine water with fruits, herbs, or spices, and let it sit for a while before drinking. The chia seeds will not only add a unique texture but also help keep you hydrated longer.

Chia seeds are not just a trendy health food; they are a functional addition to our diets that can significantly enhance hydration. With their unique ability to absorb water, provide essential minerals, and sustain energy,chia seeds are a valuable tool in the quest for optimal hydration.

Conclusion

Congratulations on reaching the end of "Constipation-Free Living: A 30-Day Chia Seed Cleanse"! We hope this journey has empowered you with valuable knowledge and practical tools to enhance your digestive health. By incorporating chia seeds into your daily routine, you've not only embraced a nutrient-rich superfood but also taken significant steps towards alleviating constipation and promoting overall well-being.

Over the past 30 days, you've learned how to harness the incredible benefits of chia seeds—from their unique ability to absorb water and create a gel-like consistency, which aids in digestion, to their rich content of fiber, omega-3 fatty acids, and essential nutrients. You now understand the importance of staying hydrated, maintaining a balanced diet, and cultivating healthy habits that contribute to a thriving digestive system.

Remember, the principles you've adopted during this cleanse are not just a temporary fix but can be integrated into your long-term lifestyle. As you continue your journey to a healthier gut, consider experimenting with different chia seed recipes, exploring additional fiber sources, and listening to your body's needs. Your awareness and commitment to your digestive health are vital.

We encourage you to share your experiences with friends, family, or a community that values health and wellness. Your journey may inspire others to explore natural solutions for their own digestive challenges.

Thank you for choosing "Constipation-Free Living" as your guide. May your newfound knowledge bring you comfort, vitality, and an enduring sense of well-being. Here's to a future filled with ease, wellness, and constipation-free living!

Biography

Alice's journey began with her own struggles with constipation, which led her to delve deep into the science of gut health. Through rigorous research and experimentation, she discovered the incredible benefits of chia seeds and a holistic approach to wellness. Her book is a culmination of her extensive knowledge, practical tips, and personal anecdotes, all aimed at helping readers achieve optimal digestive health.

Beyond her professional expertise, Alice is an avid advocate for natural living. She enjoys experimenting with new superfoods, practicing yoga, and sharing her wellness journey with her community. Her enthusiasm for health and wellness is contagious, inspiring countless individuals to take charge of their digestive health and live their best lives.

Alice Klayn's book is not just a guide—it's an invitation to embark on a life-changing journey toward better health and well-being. Through her engaging writing and deep understanding of the topic, Alice empowers her readers to embrace the power of gut health and transform their lives from the inside out.

Glossary: chia seeds for constipation

Chia Seeds

Definition: Chia seeds (Salvia hispanica) are tiny black or white seeds derived from the flowering plant native to Mexico and Guatemala. They are known for their high nutrient content, including omega-3 fatty acids, protein, fiber, and various essential minerals.

Key Terms

Fiber: A type of carbohydrate that the body cannot digest. It plays a crucial role in digestive health by promoting regular bowel movements and preventing constipation. Chia seeds are particularly high in soluble fiber, which absorbs water and forms a gel-like substance in the gut.

Hydrophilic: The property of a substance (like chia seeds) that allows it to absorb water. When soaked in water, chia seeds can expand to several times their original size, creating a gelatinous texture that helps bulk up stool and facilitate its passage through the intestines.

Bulk-forming Laxative: A natural substance that helps create bulk in the stool, promoting regular bowel movements. Chia seeds act as a bulk-forming laxative by expanding in the digestive tract when they absorb water.

Omega-3 Fatty Acids: Essential fats that the body cannot produce on its own. They are crucial for overall health, supporting heart health, reducing inflammation, and potentially improving digestive health.Chia seeds are one of the richest plant sources of omega-3s.

Prebiotics: Non-digestible fibers that serve as food for beneficial gut bacteria. Chia seeds can act as prebiotics, promoting a healthy gut microbiome, which may indirectly help alleviate constipation by improving overall digestive function.

Mechanism of Action

Chia seeds alleviate constipation through several mechanisms:

Water Absorption: When consumed, chia seeds absorb water and expand, thereby increasing stool bulk and promoting regular bowel movements. This can help soften the stool, making it easier to pass.

Gel Formation: The soluble fiber in chia seeds forms a gel-like substance in the gut, which can help maintain intestinal hydration and prevent hard stools.

Gut Health: By acting as prebiotics, chia seeds enhance the growth of beneficial gut bacteria, which can improve overall digestive health and aid in regular bowel function.

Nutritional Content: Chia seeds are not only high in fiber but also packed with nutrients that support digestive health. Their omega-3 fatty acids can help reduce inflammation in the gut, potentially leading to a healthier digestive tract.

Practical Usage

How to Incorporate Chia Seeds:

Soaking: To maximize their benefits, chia seeds should be soaked in water or another liquid (like juice or yogurt) for at least 30 minutes before consumption. This allows them to expand and form a gel-like consistency.

Smoothies: Add a tablespoon of soaked chia seeds to your morning smoothie for a nutritious boost.

Puddings: Chia seed pudding is a popular dish where chia seeds are mixed with milk (dairy or plant-based) and left to sit overnight, creating a creamy, fiber-rich dessert.

Baking: Substitute chia seeds for eggs in recipes, using a ratio of one tablespoon of chia seeds mixed with three tablespoons of water to replace one egg.